Philip Dunn a married man with three childen was born in 1935. He has had a variety of occupations; leaving school at 15 he joined HMS GANGES and spent 10 years in the Royal Navy serving on a range of ships from aircraft carriers to minesweepers. This was followed by two years at the Government Communications Headquarters in Cheltenham. In 1962 he left GCHQ to work for the Ministry of Defence in Cyprus for 6 years; it was here he acquired his first taste of journalism writing for the English language Cyprus Mail, where he had a regular TV column and contributed science articles. On returning to the UK he started his own Insurance Brokerage which he built up over the next 27 years.

In 1994 he was diagnosed with BPH, and found that substantial information was not readily available to the public. Much to his surprise he found that there was no help group for this serious medical condition, so he formed one. The work involved soon encroached on his insurance business to the extent that he had to make a decision of closing one of them down. The PHA (Prostate Help Association), by now a registered charity, won and he sold his insurance business.

Philip now works full time for the Association and has not yet regretted the decision !!

This book is dedicated to my wife, for without her encouragement and painstaking work on my countless drafts this book would never have seen the light of day.

Grateful thanks are also extended to Mark for interest above and beyond, to Nigel for coming at things from a different angle plus excellent suggestions and to Paula and Ron for genuine help.

PROSTATE CANCER

What Every Man Should Know About
The Latest Tests, Treatments and
Possible Prevention.

Philip Dunn

Ostrich Publishing

Published by Ostrich Publishing.
Langworth,
Lincoln, LN3 5DF.

© Philip Dunn 1996

Philip Dunn asserts the moral right to be identified as the author of this work.

First published in Great Britain in 1996

All rights reserved. No part of this book may be reproduced in anyway whatsoever without written permission except in the case of brief quotations embodied in critical articles and reviews.

ISBN 0 9527 3440 0

Every effort has been made to ensure the accuracy of the contents of this book.
Readers are advised that on no account should any comment herein be treated as a substitute for qualified medical advice.
You are advised to always consult a qualified medical practitioner.
Neither the author nor the publisher can be held responsible for any loss or claim arising out of the use, or misuse of this book, or failure to take medical advice.

A Catalogue record for this book is available from the British Library

Printed by The Book Factory
35/37 Queensland Rd., London N7 7AH.

CONTENTS

Chapter.   Page

    Introduction.   2
1 Basics.   7
2 Prostate Cancer, why me ?   11
3 Symptoms and tests.   15
4 Staging & Grading.   25
5 Gently does it.   28
6 Non-drug related treatment options.   32
7 Drug/hormone related treatments.   39
8 Pain treatment and care.   45
9 Prevention ?   51
10 The alternative view.   60
11 Still unsure ?   66
12 Other types of prostate tumours.   68
13 Paragraphs to ponder.   70

Appendix   75
Helpful addresses.   78
Useful books to read.   87
Letters.   88
INDEX.   93

Note.. See the back pages for a 'Cut Out' 'Bookmark' This will help you to understand some of the terminology.

INTRODUCTION

This book is written for men who have just been diagnosed with prostate cancer and for those who have been on treatments for months but can find no information as to what is happening today or what is going to happen in the future. It is also written for the men who are looking into the future and wish to see if there are any steps that can be taken to reduce the chances of having to face what their fathers or brothers are facing today.

The purpose of this book is to direct & guide you along paths you can follow. It outlines the current tests and those that will be available soon. It describes tests you should be having as opposed to those you may be offered.

Try not to be put off by any medical jargon you see in the text. I have tried to explain each term and abbreviation as it occurs. There is also a page on the reverse of the cover with problem words etc. listed for easy reference.

This book explains the degree of harm that the treatments available may cause your body, this will allow you to work your way up the treatment tree, and leave the most harmful as a last resort, if you have the choice. Everyone has their own opinion on what they regard as unacceptable. Just because YOU feel that you don't wish to become impotent (an inability to achieve an erection), your neighbour may not place it so high on his list.

For instance, if you have a urinary obstruction, maybe a TURAPY (see page 35) treatment will sort out the problem for you rather than a TURP (see page 33). The former has no apparent side effects whilst the latter 'can' cause long term problems, and could possibly disseminate a prostate cancer.

Remember you are moving into new areas of your life. Some of it may appear daunting, but disregard any feelings you may have that it really isn't for you; that you wish you didn't have to get involved and that you had better leave it to the experts. Let me tell you now that if you saw the letters I see every week you would not want to do that.

Your life is too precious to leave others to totally dictate its course. Hopefully this book will help you. Take each page as it comes, don't worry if you don't understand some of it. Skim through the whole book, then start again a little more slowly.

Gradually you will start to understand the meaning of words that you didn't know before and the reasons for the treatments will start to make sense. You will find that conversations you hear between the medics will be understandable. What it means is that you will slowly grow in confidence as you find you know more about your condition than the nurse and that you can have constructive discussions with your medical team.

Taking prescription drugs will mean you are accepting the possibility of suffering some side effects from the 'cure'. You read about all the possible side effects listed on the box but you don't expect to suffer from all of them, or even a small proportion. In the same way this book goes into detail about a host of problems that you may never suffer from. So treat it like the details on the box you get your tablets in. This author was determined not to produce a bland book which left out all the truth of the problem. Yorkshire born, I call a spade a spade !

Many of the letters the PHA receive deplore the medical profession for being somewhat reticent about prostate cancer. Many men have operations, and it is not until several months later that they find that the prostate operation had detected prostate cancer.

The general reaction to being told you have cancer is fear, understandably so. Judging from the letters the PHA get there is also a feeling of isolation. One gentleman mentioned he eventually pulled himself together to go to a cancer group meeting and found himself in 'an all woman breast cancer' situation. He felt somewhat inhibited in discussing his prostate condition as he did with most people he met. Indeed there are many reports of 'friends' not calling, and even family not being able to relate to the newly diagnosed cancer patient.

But by far the main concern, which can only increase the fear factor, is lack of knowledge. What tests ? what treatments ? what side effects ? how long ?. So now you have taken the first step to reduce the fear. Just by reading this book you will be able to negate a lot of it because you will have the answer to all those questions just posed.

At the back of the book are letters from men and their wives. I hope some of their comments will make you realise how important it is to take charge and remain in charge of your life.

Philip Dunn.

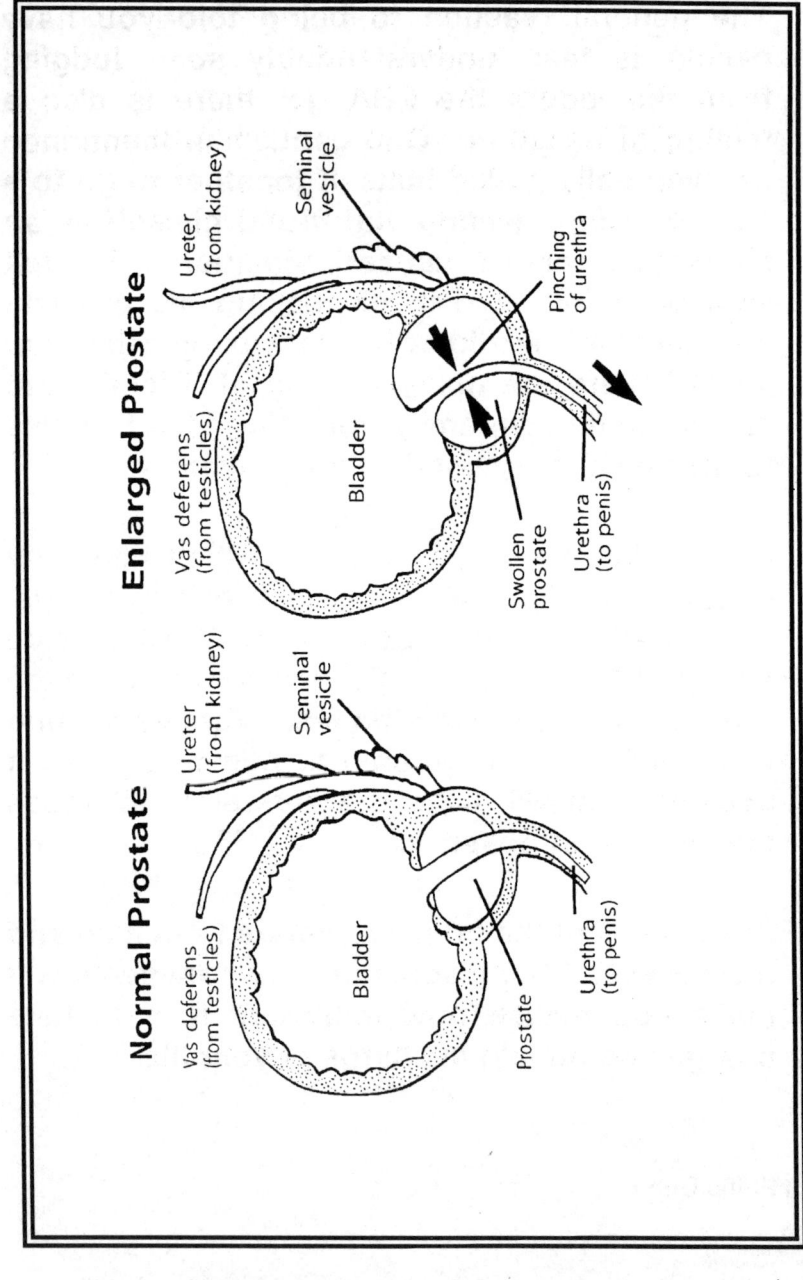

CHAPTER ONE

BASICS.

Only men have a prostate gland and are susceptible to cancer of the prostate. The prostate gland is an important part of the male urogenital system. It is located just below the bladder and is made up of many small glands which secrete a fluid into the semen before it is ejaculated. This fluid is thought to nourish the sperm in some way, but its exact function is still unknown. The normal size of a prostate in a young man is about the size of a walnut. In the majority of men the gland increases in size as we age. It expands both outward and inward and can eventually squeeze the passageway in the prostate centre causing the urine flow to weaken.

The centre of the prostate has an opening top to bottom, through which the sperm travel as too does the urine when it is being expelled from the bladder. There are two main sphincter muscles, one at the juncture of the bladder and the prostate, this set closes off to prevent sperm being ejaculated backwards into the bladder and to prevent urine being mixed with semen. These muscles are sometimes destroyed or damaged during a TURP (**Trans-Urethral Resection of the Prostate**) and it is this destruction which causes the major side effect of the operation, i.e. retrograde ejaculation. The sperm moves back into the bladder rather than being pushed down the urethra and out through the penis. The sperm is subsequently expelled (voided) on the next visit to the toilet. The second set of muscles are BELOW the prostate.

Because the prostate is located within your body it is difficult to check physically, although a GP can feel a portion of the prostate by inserting a gloved finger into the rectum. This procedure is called a DRE (**Digital Rectal Examination**) and is one method of checking to diagnose prostate cancer.

BENIGN OR MALIGNANT ?

The PHA **(Prostate Help Association)** often get letters from men who believe that benign enlargement **(BPH) (Benign Prostatic Hyperplasia)** is the pre-cursor to a full blown malignant cancer. Thankfully this isn't so otherwise the death rate from prostate cancer would be of plague proportions. The cells of the prostate reproduce like all cells by dividing in an orderly manner, this allows for the replacement and repair of the prostate tissue. Malfunction of this normality allows the cells to grow in an uncontrolled manner, this causes the increase in size of the prostate.

Benign enlargement, **(BPH)** starts its growth in the centre of the prostate and gradually works outwards, often compressing the urethra (the urine passageway) as it grows. Although uncontrolled to a degree, such cell growth is still centred within the localised area of the prostate and will not spread out of this area.

Ninety five per cent of prostate cancers begin in the glands of the prostate and are known as glandular cancers **(adenocarcinomas).** Some of the others start from the connective tissue close to or around the prostate, whilst the rest start in the ducts within the prostate. It is also possible for cancer to be spread to the prostate from the bladder. A malignant growth, prostate gland cancer, often begins at the outer portion of the gland. This means that even after a prostate resection operation, as the outer 'skin' of the gland is left intact there is still an area for the prostate cancer to begin to grow. These tumours can spread from the prostate to nearby areas, and in some cases can be carried by the bloodstream or by the lymphatic system to other areas of the body and become established there. The first spread is normally detected in the lymph nodes close to the prostate. The cancer can eventually move to most areas of the body.

Survival of a man with a prostate cancer is related directly to the growth of the cancer. Confined to the prostate gland the disease is thought to be curable. Once spread outside the prostate gland then the disease is not normally curable although average survival can be some 5 years. If the cancer has spread to other distant organs then there is no known cure at this time and the average survival is from one to three years. Having said that much longer survival periods have been known. It should also be pointed out that diagnostic techniques are not 100% accurate, this means that a diagnosis of a cancer confined to the prostate gland is not necessarily cast iron 100% reliable advice.

So bearing that in mind and the fact that we all have to die at some point in time, if you are told you have a cancer it does not necessarily mean an early death sentence. Wrong diagnosis, and the fact that prostate cancer can be a very slow growing cancer, plus the treatments now available all mean that nothing is going to happen to take your breath away today.

If the diagnosis does point to a serious situation you will feel completely disorientated. You may even feel that your condition is a retribution from the gods for misdemeanours in your early life, forget it, they have better things to do with their time. I trust that this book and the help telephone numbers and addresses at the back of the book will enable you to make a start to ensure that your quality of life is not lowered by your disease.

When this book says take charge of your life it does not mean you have to bully your way forward. What it means is that you need to increase the knowledge and understanding you have of prostate cancer so that you are no longer placed in a position of total dependence on your medics because of your 'ignorance' (that isn't meant to say that you are stupid, but means you just haven't had the facts put in front of you yet !!)

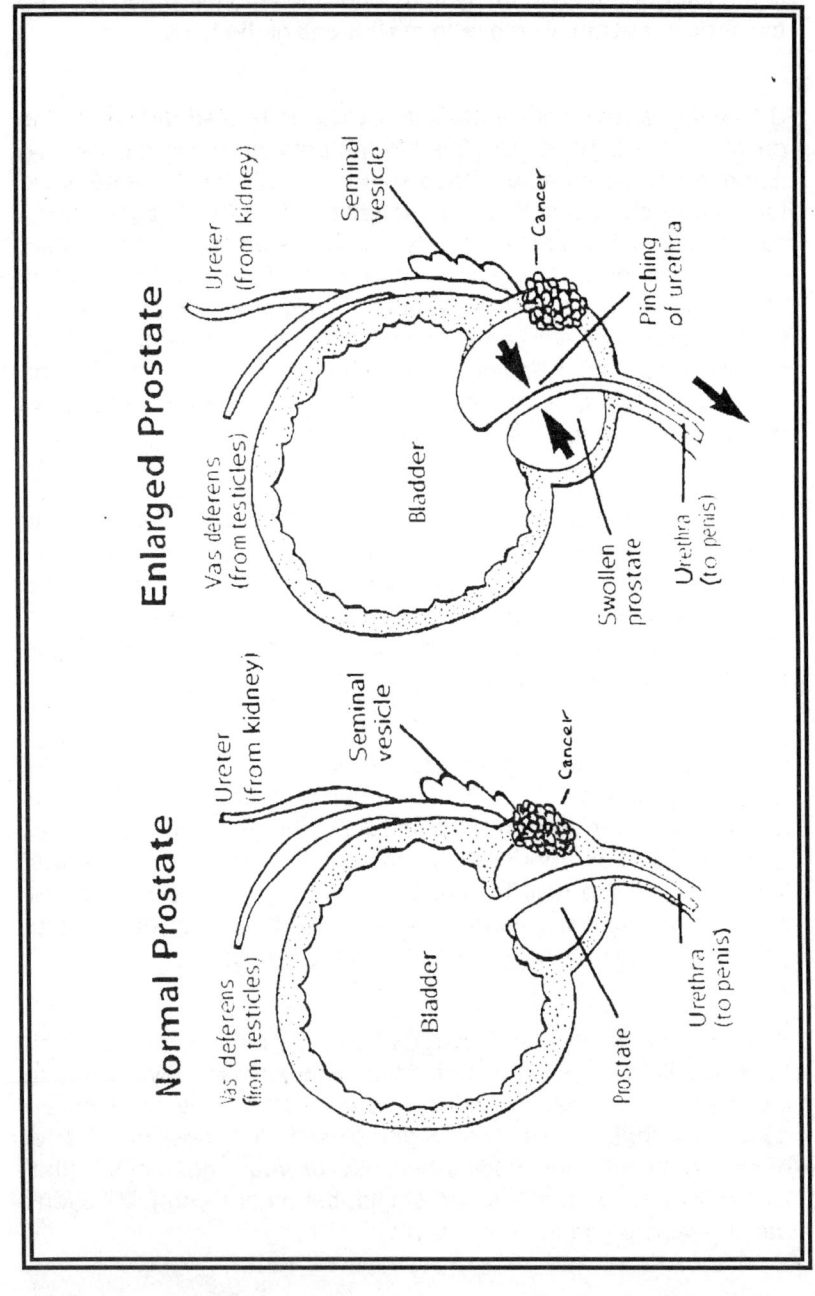

CHAPTER TWO

PROSTATE CANCER, "WHY ME?"

No one knows why you. Not a great deal of money is spent in this country on research so it will probably be a breakthrough in the USA which will answer that question. What is known is that certain things can increase your chances of getting this disease. Some old wives tales can be hit on the head. There is no evidence that venereal disease or sexual activity causes prostate cancer, and likewise no evidence that a partner can catch a cancer through sexual contact. Recent comment in regard to a vasectomy operation giving a man an increased risk of prostate cancer have also not been shown to be accurate.

* **AGE FACTOR.** As you grow older the chances of contracting prostate cancer increases. With an increasing older population this cancer is expected to become the largest cause of death in the male. Although the majority of those diagnosed are well into their 60's and over, the PHA **(Prostate Help Association)** knows from the letters it receives that many men below the age of 50 have succumbed.

* **FAMILY CONNECTION.** You should be aware that if your male relations, brothers, father, uncles etc., have had a prostate cancer then you have an increased risk. This does not mean you will get prostate cancer, but that you are in a higher risk category. It therefore makes good sense if you are in that category to think very seriously about annual checks from your GP, this means a PSA, a DRE, & a TRUS, (see from page 17 on) to ensure that your prostate remains clear of any problems. In such a situation the PHA would advise to start checks from the age of 45 at least. It is possible that before too long a

scientist will isolate a gene, which indicates a propensity for the disease, this would forewarn anyone who was in the firing line.

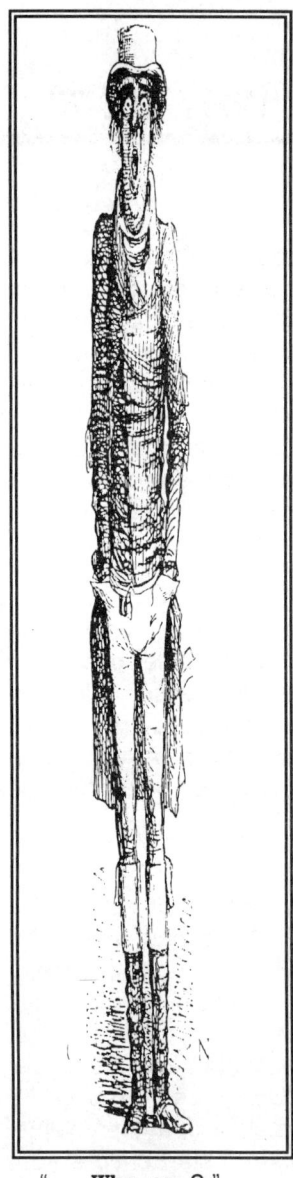

" Why me ? "

* **RACIAL** . African American men are at the top of the high risk ladder, while Asian men are on the lowest rung, yet only if they remain in their own country and do not pursue a Western life style. Once in the USA, for instance, a Japanese man will begin to face similar risks to any other American. However there has been some comment that it takes a generation for this to happen. The Chinese have one twentieth the cancer rate of men in the UK, whilst Swedes have more than double the rate. Regrettably the reasons for these differences are not known although there are some theories mainly in connection with food intake.

* **DIET**. Prostate cancer and heart disease in Asian countries are low compared to Western countries. Asians, until recently, have had a low red meat/high vegetable diet. Studies around the world have shown a **consistent** amount of microscopic cancers in men who have died accidentally. Yet deaths from prostate cancer in Western countries are much higher. For instance, the death rate in Japan is less than a quarter of the US rate. It was put down to genetics, but a study of immigrants showed that prostate cancers diagnosed rose even in first generation immigrants. Recent figures

indicate that Japanese, in Japan, living in urban areas are increasing their red meat/high fat consumption and causing a rise in prostate cancer rates. This compares with no increase in rural areas where there is still a low red meat/low fat diet.

* **CANCER EXPLOSION.** If we set aside the fact that an aging population will in itself produce more cancers, there is some evidence that there are not necessarily more prostate cancers in the population, just a lot more being found because of new testing methods. As there is also a good case for not treating many prostate cancers (if they are small and non aggressive,) you would do well to ignore the tabloid press when it uses headlines to shock. Beware the scalpel and any other treatment until you have a well balanced view of your cancer and of the varied treatments available to you.

* **TESTOSTERONE.** There is no certainty as to the cause of prostate cancer. One theory is that it might be linked to testosterone; a male hormone. It has been noted that men who have had their testicles removed before puberty very rarely get prostate cancer. Conversely it appears that body builders and men who increase their testosterone levels may have an enhanced possibility of getting the disease. One significant pointer is that Merck Pharmaceuticals are running a clinical trial with 18,000 men. They are using the drug Proscar, (finasteride), in a clinical study to see if regular use can reduce the risk of prostate cancer. Proscar inhibits the production of DHT (dihydrotestosterone), which is converted from testosterone. DHT is thought to be the cause of BPH. **(Benign Prostatic Hyperplasia).**

DOES EVERY MAN GET PROSTATE CANCER ?

The answer to that is almost every man will if they live long enough. It seems that 90% of men over 90 will have some sign of prostate cancer. But the small areas (foci) of cancer found in most men will not give them any problem, and without some form of test they would never know that they had the foci at all.

After post-mortems, following an accidental death, men in their 50's have been shown to have similar foci. It also appears that on average all men around the world have a similar incidence of foci and that includes the Far East and the West. But what is most important to bear in mind is that having a prostate cancer and death being caused by that prostate cancer is not a foregone conclusion. **More men die WITH prostate cancer than OF it.**

So you are strongly advised to beware of being drawn into a cycle of medical treatments. Even before you go to your GP for a DRE (**Digital Rectal Examination**), or a PSA (**Prostate Specific Antigen**) test, you would be well advised to read up on the subject and gain knowledge, for with that knowledge will come confidence and the ability to make important decisions about your own future. Even if you are diagnosed with prostate cancer it is important to know that it may be classed as non-aggressive; a latent cancer. Such a cancer will probably never give you any cause for concern apart from the psychological worry you could give yourself because you know it is there. So discuss with your GP or Specialist the options, be particularly aware of **'watchful waiting'**, that does not mean 'doing nothing', it means keeping a close eye on the problem. But most beneficial of all, it means you are not going to subject your body to the trauma of drugs, radiotherapy, or surgery, which may never be needed.

Watchful waiting does not apply if you are diagnosed with an aggressive cancer, which gives you a very high PSA reading and may have metastasized, **(Passed/Spread)** into the bone.

CHAPTER THREE

SYMPTOMS AND TESTS.

Currently there is not a self testing kit for prostate cancer, although a DIY PSA test is scheduled. What there can be are signs, although sadly it is true that some men have prostate cancer with no outward signs at all until the disease is well advanced.

National screening for prostate cancer is called for from some quarters, but does not meet with universal approval. Once some of the tests, which are written about later in this book, become available then screening possibly becomes worth the cost involved, but having said that there is currently no evidence that treatment of a prostate cancer, once diagnosed by screening, will actually prolong the patients life. This is very similar to lung cancer; another cancer with no national screening programme.

With over two million men in the UK having some form of prostate problem and over 300,000 thought to visit their GP every year for prostate consultations, there is a growing fear amongst a large section of the medical profession in regard to testing.

As the public become more aware of prostate cancer and the PSA test, more men are asking for a check up. This is leading to the diagnosis of more and more early prostate cancers. Reginald Hall, a consultant at the Freeman Hospital in Newcastle, said in November 1995, "early prostate cancer poses a considerable dilemma for doctors and patients because it is not clear what to do. We don't know how to pick out those that will progress and those that we should leave alone".

It is claimed that national screening here in the UK would find 150,000 prostate cancers. In the USA the policy is to operate as soon as possible after diagnosis to ensure the cancer has no chance of spreading. Here in the UK the policy of 'watch & wait' is much more favourably looked upon. Many would cynically say this is because of the cost to the nation. At a conference in Paris, Mr Hall explained "If all men between 50 and 70 had a PSA test , a biopsy and surgery, the cost to the NHS would be £450 million" Yet, there is another side to that.

There is no proof that an early operation actually prolongs the life of a man diagnosed with a cancer. A man so diagnosed and demanding the surgical route is perhaps letting cold fear take over from logical thought.

Mr Hall said he, "would remove prostates with early cancer if the man insisted. We leave the choice to the man and his wife. We have no scientific or statistical facts to say which is best for him, it is a horrible situation to be in. Patients get very upset because they expect doctors to know what is best for them, but we have to be honest and say that we don't know."

Incidentally the above figures are suspect, in that if all men between 50-70 initially had a PSA and DRE test many would be ruled out of any further testing. Of the remainder who then went on to a biopsy, once again many of those would be ruled out, and no surgery would be required. So there is no way that all men between 50-70 would require a test, a biopsy and surgery. This means of course that the figure of £450 million has no basis in fact. Yet you can be sure that in the months ahead journalists and possibly even government health ministers will be quoting it as if it is authoritative.

What is known with is that the majority of the estimated 150,000 men diagnosed with prostate cancer would never die from the cancer found. I repeat "It is a fact that more men die **with** prostate cancer than die **of** it." This is because prostate cancer, in many cases, is very slow growing. Without screening a man could live out his life with no worry and no problem from the small cancer cells in his body, so prompt surgical action is not necessarily the answer. The problem with taking the surgical route is that a man ramps up his chances of spoiling his retirement years. The operation not only has a mortality risk but can also cause impotence, infertility, incontinence and even a possibility of cancer spread.

So just what are the symptoms of prostate cancer ?

* A slow urine flow rate, and/or trips to the bathroom at night, are all signs of possible urinary obstruction.

* Multiple visits to the bathroom during the day over and above what was the norm six months or a year ago.

* Tiredness, loss of appetite and weight loss.

* Blood in the urine or sperm.

* Bone pain (this could be from secondary tumours).

Some of these symptoms equate to BPH benign prostate growth, so do not automatically assume you have a prostate cancer because you are making frequent trips to the bathroom for instance. You are recommended to pay a visit to your GP for a check up.

I hate to say this, but just because you do not have the above symptoms does not mean you do not have prostate cancer. Some cancers can proceed to a very advanced state before any apparent symptoms appear.

How will your GP/Specialist check your prostate for BPH or a possible prostate cancer ?

There are several tests and you should be aware that you should in no way rely solely on any one test..

* **URINE ANALYSIS.** Routine analysis of a urine sample to look for traces of blood or infection in the urine, plus checks on liver and kidney function.

* **DRE. Digital Rectal Examination.** This is a gloved index finger, well lubricated, inserted into the rectal passageway. Just inside and toward the front of the body and just behind the

internal rectal wall lies the prostate gland. The GP can feel the gland through the wall. The surface of the gland should feel smooth, irregularities could signal cancer growth, although it could be a stone. A report in the BMJ (British Medical Journal) in 1994 indicated that DRE screening was only accurate in 30-40% of cases.

Seventy-five percent of GP's claim to find it difficult to differentiate between BPH **(Benign prostatic hyperplasia)** (an enlarged prostate) and prostate cancer whilst performing a DRE. What is of more concern is that some 50% feel that they have not had adequate training in diagnosis.

Small tumours should feel like a small pea, whereas an advanced prostate cancer would produce the feel of a hard irregular mass. This contrasts with a normal prostate which should be smooth and even to the touch.

* **PSA. Prostate Specific Antigen.** For the technically-minded, PSA is a glycoprotein which causes the seminal coagulant to liquefy. The amount of PSA is related more or less to the size of the prostate or cancer and is therefore a useful measure of the progression of prostate disease. In strictly numerical terms, however, if the level is raised above 4.0 this could indicate that a cancer is present. This is a test on a sample of blood and takes about 7 days for a result.

Because it has always been understood that an examination of the prostate may effect a PSA reading your GP should take a blood sample, from your arm, **before** doing the DRE. Mr Roger Kirby, Consultant Urologist, in an article in Pulse May 1995 indicated that a DRE does not raise PSA levels. I have seen no follow up advice on this however. He also mentions that retrospective studies of stored serum samples suggest that the PSA levels begin to rise as much as 10 years before clinical diagnoses. Could this have a connection with PIN ? **(prostatic intraepithelial neoplasia)** (see page 69).

Recommendations are that as the PSA level in a healthy man over the age of 40 is from 0-4ng/ml, **(Nanograms per millilitre, a nanogram is one thousandth of a millionth of a gram)** a reading of over 4ng/ml should be referred for further investigation. However a PSA reading can be increased by other factors apart from prostate cancer. Each extra gram of BPH tissue can increase the PSA by 0.3ng/ml. So an enlarged prostate can push the PSA reading above 4ng/ml. The older you are the higher your PSA is likely to be. It is thought that PSA can increase by some 3.2 % per year in a healthy older male. This means that in the USA PSA guide lines are currently 2.5ng/ml for men from 40 to 49, (not the 4ng/ml as mentioned above) 3.5ng/ml between 50-59, 4.5ng/ml between 60-69 and 6.5ng/ml from 70-79. An inflamed prostate can also raise levels, so as Corporal Jones would tell you, "Don't Panic" if you have a PSA test and it appears high. Any of the factors above may be the reason, or it could just be an incorrect assessment. A second reading is to be recommended before any major investigation if the first reading is high. Remember a PSA velocity, its year by year increase, is very useful. As a cancer grows faster than BPH, a man with cancer is likely to have a higher year by year change than a man with BPH alone. Cancer cells incidently produce 15 times more PSA than true prostate cells.

A further comment on PSA is in regard to the drug Proscar (finasteride). This is normally a treatment for BPH, (see later comment on its use as a possible cancer preventative), however, it is known to lower the PSA level, so be sure that the medical staff who take your blood sample know you are taking Proscar so that they can take this into consideration.

It is also worth noting that the PSA can reach different levels dependent upon the type of cancer treatment the patient is having. So it is no good comparing your PSA levels with your colleague if he is on a different treatment.

RAD Magazine in January 1995 reported on a long term study of almost 1,000 men with prostate cancer in the USA. The study, which covered treatments given over a period from 1969 to 1991, showed that levels of PSA gave a good indicator of survival times.

For instance, levels up to 10ng/mg gave a 75%, or higher, probability of 5 to 10 years survival compared to lower percentage survival rates for higher levels. In other words if you have a cancer with a PSA level of 10ng/mg or lower you have at least a 75% chance of living 5 to 10 years. If the PSA level is higher then that chance is below 75%.

Another study, once again in the USA, has shown that there are in fact two types of PSA to be measured. The new key one is known as a measure of free floating PSA. Tests have indicated that men with a free floating PSA below 20% had a higher chance of having cancer than those with a free floating PSA above 20%. A national trial has begun (in the USA) using some 12,000 patients to confirm the original study. In practical terms, using this test would mean that some 70% of men, who are currently shown to need biopsies, would no longer need them for the new test would rule them out. This is not only a cost saving but think of the 'worry saving' to the men as well.

Ask your GP/Specialist, if you are going for your first check-up, if this test is available. A recent article by Dr. A Milford-Ward, of the Northern General Hospital, Sheffield, discussing free floating PSA, apparently there are a number of 'kits', presumably produced by different companies. A problem appeared to be in 1994 that there was not a standardisation between the companies. At least it means that your medical team should know what you mean when you ask for a 'free' PSA check. Hopefully the answer will **not** be that it's free on the NHS !

One further bout of confusion within the medical profession occurred in November of 1995 when the BMJ (British Medical Journal) sent out a press release to every major news agency, indeed the PHA had phone calls for comment from both Sky News and from the BBC TV. Although the PHA spokesman attempted to explain that the article was ambiguous to say the least, this was not the line that the journalist wanted and was ignored. The BMJ press release stated that **"the PSA test could predict prostate cancer accurately."** Odd that, on page 1178 of the November issue of the Lancet Jonathan Waxman, an Oncologist, stated **"the comparative failure of PSA as a diagnostic test was** shown in 366 men who developed prostate cancer during participation in a Physicians Health Study."

The bad thing about the left hand not knowing what the right hand is doing was that the BBC, ITV, Sky News and the major national newspapers all had an item in regard to the BMJ press release saying that the PSA test could accurately predict prostate cancer. What is the man in the street to make of his GP's response, depending upon which medical paper the GP reads, or of the government attitude, for they refuse to implement a national screening programme because there is no robust cancer test yet ?

Rising PSA levels after treatments are indicative of treatment failures.

* **PAP. Prostatic Acid Phosphatase**. PAP levels are elevated if a tumour has spread to the bone. This is an **old test** and not 100% accurate. It should not be used in place of a PSA test when you go for your first check up.

* **TRUS.   Trans-Rectal Ultra Sound**. An Ultrasound machine passes sound waves through the body and create an image on a screen. To enable the image to be seen more clearly the room is darkened. The majority of ultra sound tests are carried out by passing a device across the abdomen. It is a simple and painless procedure. It is recommended you ask for a **transrectal ultrasound**, because as the probe is nearer to the prostate, [the device is inserted in the rectal passage], it will give a better image and allow the operator to see any abnormalities much more clearly and accurately within the prostate gland. Have no fear, the probe is well lubricated and the whole procedure a non- event compared to any trauma you can build up in your mind over the weeks prior to your appointment. A report in The Practitioner magazine in June 1992 advised that use of TRUS doubled the detection rate of prostate cancer. The operator will take the opportunity to check the amount of urine which is failing to leave the bladder so you will be asked to top up with liquid prior to the test. After the bladder has been measured you leave the room and visit a nearby toilet, then return and the amount of residual liquid can be measured. This test could take approx 15 minutes.

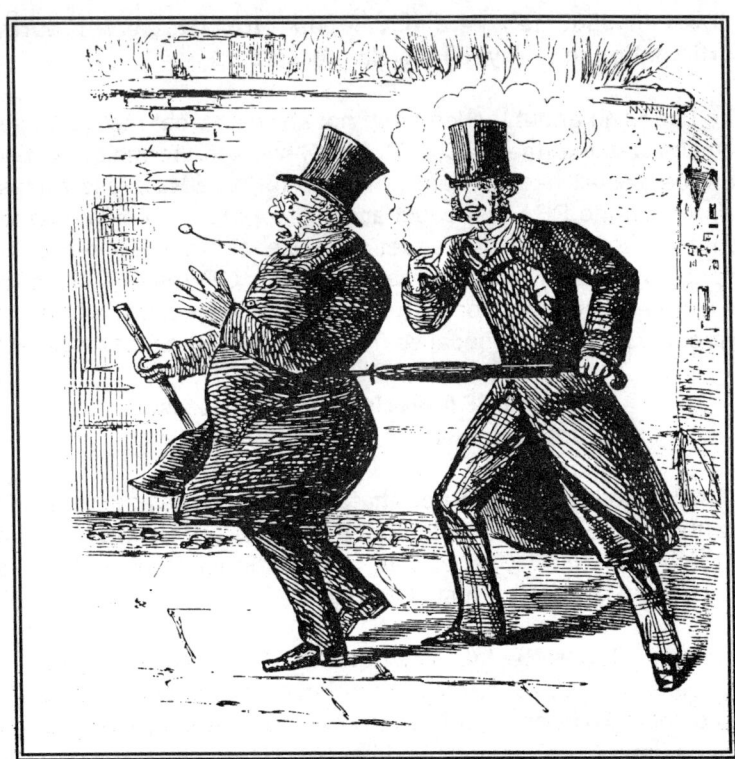

"Biopsy. A thin needle inserted into the prostate tissue"

* **CYSTOSCOPY.** The passing of a small viewing tube through the urethra to view the prostate and also the bladder if necessary.

* **BIOPSY.** A thin needle inserted, (normally under local anaesthetic) into the prostate tissue via the back passage. This procedure takes samples of prostate tissue to examine for cancer cells and can take a little longer than 30 mins, but should not be longer than one hour. There is a chance of infection due to the proximity of the prostate to the rectum and its contents. You should ensure that you are given antibiotics to reduce this possibility.

More research from the USA into the analysis of biopsy samples indicates that such analysis can apparently predict the aggressiveness of prostate cancer. So far evidence has not been found that such analysis of samples are carried out in the UK. A report in the RAD magazine in September 1995 said that it was already an established fact that DNA analysis of tumours after removal was the best way to predict a chance of a reoccurrence or spread. The fact that an analysis of a small biopsy sample can give similar indicators must be a big plus for anyone faced with a decision as to which treatment to choose.

The technique allows for the cancer cells from the sample to be divided into two distinct groups. One called **'diploid'** and the other **'aneuploid'**. It appears that aneuploid cancers are three times more likely to reoccur, are twice as likely to spread and ten times more likely to move into the bone.

If the analysis is available in the UK then a patient is able to stand on firmer ground when choosing between 'watchful waiting' or a less aggressive treatment. As at this time, (December 1995), further studies are being carried out to validate the initial results, but by the time you are reading this is it will be worth asking for your biopsy sample to be sent to a major centre for such analysis. The estimated cost for such an analysis in the USA is put at some £50 maximum. Not too expensive, if the NHS is not forthcoming, if it means it gives you extra information, which will allow you to make a positive decision between radical or non-radical treatments.

* **CT. Computerised Tomography.** This scanning system is best at checking for enlargement of the lymph nodes.. Most of us are familiar with the TV images of side or end views of the body or brain. This system allows a cross section of each portion of the body scanned to be viewed on a TV screen.

* **MR (I). Magnetic Resonance Imaging**. This scanning system uses a magnetic field to create a detailed picture of your glands and bones etc. It gives a better pictures of the prostate and seminal vesicle than the CT above. However, not all men can take advantage of this screening system. Things which will cancel you out are:- if you have a heart pacemaker, have any metal fragments in your eyes, (through being a metal worker) or have had any heart valves replaced with metal valves. You will

also need to wear clothing which have no metal fastenings. Occasionally a contrast medium will be injected into a vein, not the prostate, to enhance the images. This scan should take from 30 mins to one hour.

* **FLOW RATE.** This requires you to pass urine into a funnel, the flow is checked by a computer in most cases, which provides an indication of any obstruction problems. The time it takes depends on your flow rate !

If you are involved with any of these checks and you are not sure about anything that is happening, ask, query and ensure that you are fully satisfied before you go ahead.

CHAPTER FOUR

STAGING AND GRADING.

Staging is a method of assessing the progress of the cancer according to the amount of its growth and spread. The US method is the American Urologic Association classification.

Stage 'A' The cancer is virtually undetectable by any means other than by tissue analysis.

Stage 'B' The cancer can be detected by a DRE, and is confined to the prostate gland.

Stage 'C' The cancer is spread just out from the prostate gland.

Stage.'D' The cancer has spread away from the prostate and is in other areas of the body.

Numbers can be added to the letters to further differentiate the degree of growth and spread.

A system more common in Europe is the International Union Against Cancer system. This uses the letters 'T', 'N' and 'M'.

T1 indicates a cancer undetectable except by tissue analysis.
T2 indicates a cancer confined to the prostate.
T3 indicates a cancer pushing through the skin (capsule) of the prostate.
T4 indicates a cancer which has moved into nearby areas.

N indicates problems with the lymph nodes.

M indicates metastatic problems, i.e. the cancer has spread to other areas of the body.

To these, can be added x, 0 (zero) and a,b,c, for instance :-

Tx indicates the cancer cannot be assessed.

T0 indicates no evidence of cancer.

T4a indicates a cancer which has moved into the bladder neck or external sphincter.

M1 indicates distant metastases.

M1b..indicates metastases in the bone.

Just what treatment can be expected to be suggested by a urologist to a patient set against these stages. You have read the somewhat indicisive comments by UK medics, although I am certain there are many who will have definate views. Here in the UK surgery for cancer is not the first line of attack. In the US there is much greater enthusiasm for it. Bearing this in mind here below are the sort of recommendations a patient would get from his US urologist. The staging has been changed to the European method.

T2.

If aged under 70 then radical prostatectomy would be a first choice with radiotherapy second. Aged 70-80 radiotherapy would be recommended. Over 80 years then watchful waiting with hormone treatment if the cancer becomes agressive.

T3.

Radiotherapy would be the recommendation.

M1.

Hormone treatment with orchidectomy.

Because each patient will be presenting to his medic with a varied degree of problems, there is no way that each patient

will be recommended the same treatment, the information is an indication of what could happen to Mr Smith and not a recommendation for a particular method for you to persue.

You will note there is no advice re 'watchful waiting' nor of MAB to downstage a cancer prior to either a radical prostatectomy or radiotherapy. These should certainly be part of your consideration and discussion with your medical team.

GRADING.

The most popular system is the Gleason system. This range of numbers from 2 to 10 is a method of describing the aggressive nature of the cancer. It is determined by examining the cancer cells under a microscope to check how they differ from the true prostate cell shape. A score of 4 or less should mean a normal life for the patient, whilst 5-9 would mean a cancer which can be expected to progress over time.

CHAPTER FIVE

GENTLY DOES IT.

If you are diagnosed with prostate cancer what you must **not do** is rush into a quick decision. You will probably feel you ought to have done something yesterday and that leaving it until tomorrow is far too long. You must totally ignore such feelings. Your first efforts must be directed at obtaining a second opinion, whilst at the same time gaining as much knowledge as you can about prostate cancer. You need to buy books or ask your reference library for the latest information they have on the subject.

A July 1995 report in the publication WDDTY 'What Doctors Don't Tell You' stated that in the USA .. "If a tumour is found it's automatically removed, but so far there isn't any evidence to show this approach makes you live longer."

Prostate cancer has a relatively slow rate of growth compared to other cancers in the body. This has been assessed at two and a half years for cancer within the prostate and one and a half years for metastatic cancer (that is cancer which has moved out from the prostate and into the surrounding bone).

Whilst you are getting confirmation that you have prostate cancer find out about the treatment options available. Are there any new ones which your GP/Specialist may be aware of but may not mention unless carefully questioned ? You then want to know what side effects each treatment may produce.

Attempt to contact other men who are suffering from prostate cancer or who have recovered. What did they do, was the

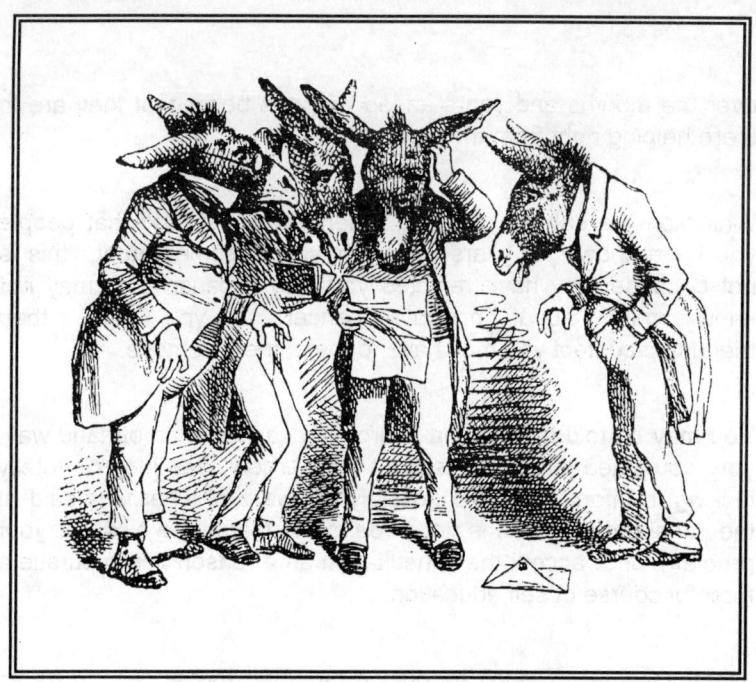

"..... have at your side the best advisors"

decision they made the right one or do they now consider another treatment would have been better, if so why? Find out if others in your position altered their diet or lifestyle, and if so has it helped them. (The addresses at the back of the book will help you).

If you make a decision based on your own knowledge of the subject then you will find it easier to live with. You managed to get through your traumatic teenage years, many didn't. You survived wars and marriage, many didn't. Regard prostate cancer as one more experience or challenge in life. Your age and current experience will allow you to confront this latest trauma with much more courage than your earlier problems in life. At least with this one there is now a vast amount of information available. There are also professional organisations such as Tenovus & Bacup (see useful addresses), who can help, most importantly you have family and/or friends. Don't hide your condition from them. They will probably never forgive you if you do and will most certainly be able to help you if you confide in them. You will need their support over the months and years ahead and it is better that they are in there helping right from the start.

Whilst on the subject of telling others, you may find that people you have known for years will avoid you to some extent, this is not because they have rejected you, but because they may not know much about prostate cancer. If you value their friendship/contact you may have to make the first move.

You may be told that you have prostate cancer in an offhand way, you could leave the consultant or surgery bewildered, totally lacking in information and possibly unaware of what was said at the consultation. This is not a reason to blame the NHS for your problem, or to accept the consultation as a reason not to pursue a forceful course of self education.

Whatever you do, don't be put off by what may appear to be an abrupt, uncaring attitude of a nurse, GP or specialist. That person is one out of a hundred and the rest are not like that. Change your GP or specialist if need be. You will need a firm ally in that department, someone who you feel able to turn to whatever the problem. So ensure that as the battle is commenced you have at your side the best advisors etc. No General ever won a battle with fellow officers he was unable to trust and rely upon. A recent book for the benefit of GP's states "Any form of treatment must be tailored to the individual patient's clinical case as well as their **informed wishes.**" 'Informed wishes', in other words, **your** requirements, following **your** decision, following full information given to **you** to enable **you** to make a logical decision.

Be aware that a British Medical Journal article in March 1993 indicated that no treatment at any stage of prostate cancer has been shown to improve survival in an adequate clinical trial. This doesn't mean that all treatments are no good, just that everything is still so new that in effect almost anyone with adequate information can have a reasoned opinion which may be correct. It may take years of clinical trials to enable the medical profession to say things like drug 'A' will give you 10 years, drug 'B' 5 years etc.

The beginning of this chapter said "don't do anything quickly", on the other hand that should not be an excuse for sitting and doing nothing, permanently ducking a decision. Do not say, "oh well, I will wait to go to see the GP the next time I'm due to collect my heart pills or some such excuse".

CHAPTER SIX
NON-DRUG RELATED TREATMENT OPTIONS

WATCHFUL WAITING. What happens is that any progression of the cancer is monitored using regular PSA and ultrasound testing methods, preferably TRUS. Many cancers do not progress, so using this option can save a man from 'aggressive' treatment which could seriously disrupt his lifestyle. A US report in January 1994 advised that 86% of patients with prostate cancer survived for 19 years after diagnosis and in two thirds of the patients the cancer had not spread. Other studies have shown that this method produces a 10 year survival rate which is almost the same as men treated with more aggressive methods. Some comment states that men over 80 are best treated by 'watchful waiting' and those under 70 with surgery or radiation. It is scratch your head time if you are between 70 and 80 as to which method you elect. Your future quality of life will depend upon the choice of treatment you have, together with your current state of health and the aggressiveness of the cancer.

* **LAPAROSCOPIC LYMPH NODE DISSECTION.** Prior to the removal of a prostate gland surgeons will check the lymph nodes to see if they contain cancer. This can be done by the use of a long thin telescope inserted through a tiny opening in the abdomen. If the lymph nodes contain cancer, then the removal of the prostate is not called for and other forms of treatment are suggested such as radiotherapy or hormone therapy.

* **RADICAL PROSTATECTOMY. (complete surgical removal of the prostate gland)** This treatment can be considered for prostate cancer which is still retained within the prostate gland. Before this operation is carried out, the surgeon will check the lymph nodes which are close to the prostate gland. These nodes are normally the first line of movement of the cancer from the prostate. Therefore if these are cancer free then treatment

can be either a radical prostatectomy, radiotherapy or both. The entire prostate is removed as well as the local lymph node groups. **Dependent upon the skill of the surgeon** the idea is to spare the adjacent nerves to preserve potency (ensure you can continue to have an erection). Regrettably some 50% of patients are rendered impotent. Incontinence is also a factor and can occur in some 5% of cases. This is a much more serious operation than the TURP and will require a longer stay in hospital. You will probably be on fluids for some time after the operation until your bowels start to work again after the trauma of the operation. A catheter could be in place for some six weeks following this operation. As you will realise after that length of time, when it is removed, some bladder training is going to be required. A Radical prostatectomy may be difficult if you have had a TURP. (See below) Many men assume that a TURP operation removes all the prostate gland, it does not. Indeed in a lot of cases the tissue left continues to grow and will cause a blockage after a few years. (Your attention is drawn to the slight possibility of dissemination as noted in the TURP treatment detail below). It must be pointed out that not all in the medical profession would agree that this is possible.

As with any major surgery there is a chance of death from heart related complications within 30 days of the operation and a patient can expect a three month recuperation period. A report in the US medical press noted it was particularly dangerous for men over 70 with a 2% death rate. Having said that, radical surgery is not carried out with as much enthusiasm in the UK as in some other countries such as the USA.

You will have to sign an authority form prior to the operation, it might be wise to ensure that you are only signing for what you have discussed with your surgeon and not for exploratory surgery.

* **TURP. (Transurethral resection of the prostate).** This operation is performed by inserting a resectoscope into the prostate via the penis. A heated wire loop then cuts away the obstructive tissue. It is normally performed to relieve obstructive symptoms caused by a growth, either benign or cancerous, which is stopping the free flow of urine. Following the operation a man may require a stay in hospital of approx. 5 days and

during half of that time he will have a catheter in place. Possible side effects of this treatment are impotence, infertility and incontinence, these could be of greater concern when the operation is carried out for BPH. However to relieve blockage caused by a cancer, at the moment, this is the recommended treatment. This surgical treatment could disseminate (spread) cancerous tissue, although this operation has been so implicated **it has not been definitely associated with such dissemination** and as mentioned earlier not all medical authorities feel that this is a fact. Hopefully the radio frequency treatment known as TURAPY may eventually be used to remove this obstructive tissue. At this moment in time you may not find a surgeon willing to use it.

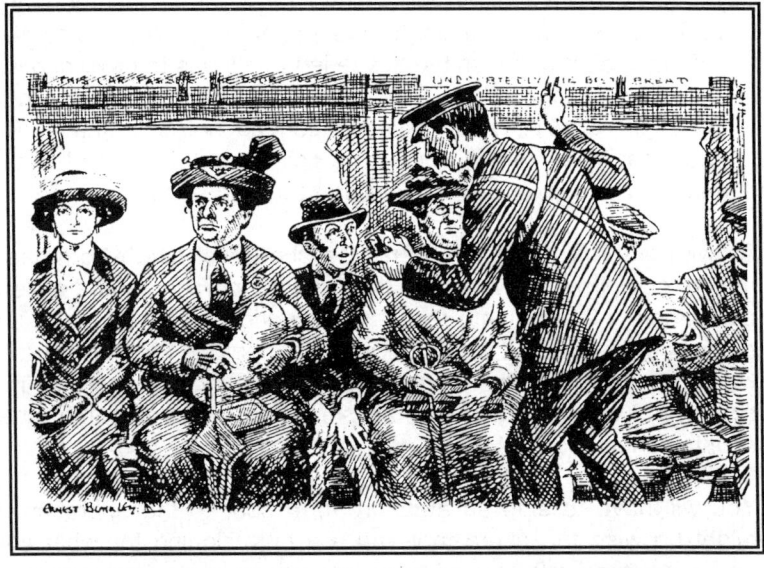

It is recommended not to drive after a radical prostatectomy or a TURP. You could use public transport instead.

Interviews with urologists in the USA on Channel 7 and CNN this year, produced very positive statements in that radical prostatectomy will cure the cancer. The UK Medical Establishment however is much less sure about this.

* **TURAPY. (Trans Urethral Ablation Prostatectomy).** This is a method of heating up the prostate tissue using radio frequency energy. Basically, this is a nonsurgical TURP, with no apparent side effects and a one hour out-patient treatment with no anaesthetic required. The results have been compared favourably with those of the 'gold standard' TURP treatment. (The medical profession in general still regard the TURP as the superior 'gold standard', BPH operation.)

* **MICROWAVE.** Although TURAPY treatment provides much higher operating temperatures with greater safety than microwave machines, it is only the latter that have been used for cancer treatment. Apparently tumour cells are much more sensitive to heat than normal cells. One study using temperatures of between 41 - 44 degrees C noticed a disappearance of the cancer in some 44 patients. The problem appears to be that it is impossible to predict if the whole of the prostate, or indeed any prostate, will heat up sufficiently to carry out the microwave treatment satisfactorily, as some prostates appear to be 'heat resistant'. Because microwaves cause hot spots it would seem that further efforts in heat treatment for prostate cancer should be done using a radio frequency machine which has a better record of tissue heating.

* **CRYOTHERAPY.** This was a technique used as a treatment for BPH. but is now used for prostate cancer. For BPH the route was via the urethra into the prostate, for prostate cancer probes are inserted into the prostate through the area between the anus and the scrotum. Once in place liquid nitrogen is fed into the probes which drop the treatment area to an extremely low temperature. Transrectal ultrasound allows the probes to be located exactly in position and incidentally allows a view of the formation of the ice front as it moves out from the probe tip. This means that the freezing can be stopped immediately the ice front nears the rectal wall. The idea is that this freezing kills off the cancer cells, as well as destroying almost all the tissue in the prostate. This treatment is not well documented or widespread, clinical feed back on the results is not available.

* **HIFU. (High-Intensity Focused Ultrasound).** This is not to be confused with the ultrasound machine, which allows an operator

to view the interior organs of the body. These machines allow a focused point of energy to an internal part of the body without any injury to any of the intervening body parts. The tissue at the focal point is ablated (destroyed). Aided by a computer the focal point can be guided to destroy selected areas of tissue. These machines have not as yet been used for the treatment of cancer but have been used for the treatment of BPH.

* **RADIOTHERAPY.** This is the use of high energy rays to kill cancer cells and could cure the prostate cancer condition if treatment is given whilst the cancer is still in the prostate capsule. The target site will not only be the prostate but also the lymph nodes which lie close to the prostate. Cancer cells are more sensitive to the treatment than normal cells so the radiotherapy kills them. You can expect a daily treatment lasting over a period of some six weeks, so you will need to travel daily to your hospital, although you will get breaks at weekends. Show an interest from the beginning. Find out what the 'dose' is you will be getting, ask to see how this is set up on the machine. If you find that you are being treated with an audience of trainees, object, nothing flusters an operator more than having someone looking over their shoulder. The last thing you want is a flustered operator ! Your body may have markings on it so that the radiographer can align the machine, so these should not be removed.

The treatment is painless. Many men experience virtually no side effects whilst they are having their treatment. Those that do mention tiredness, nausea, some diarrhoea, bladder instability and hair loss in the general area of the treatment. There is also a 25% chance you will become impotent over time and some patients develop radiation cystitis. If you feel tired, plan to take things a little easier for the period of your treatment. If you are still at work see if you can temporarily reduce your work hours.

Some men feel nauseous at the beginning of the treatment, there are many techniques to help you. Physco-therapists can teach you to overcome your feelings, relaxation methods which can allow you to set aside the nausea and of course acupuncture should be given some consideration. If these techniques fail your GP may prescribe a drug to help. It is possible that some foods, such as high fibre vegetables, and fruit etc. may need to be avoided. You are also recommended to drink as much liquid as you can, but not alcohol as this could make your problems worse. Your stomach may be upset, so eating smaller amounts on a more regular basis would probably help. If all else fails there is the high calorie food 'Complan' you can try.

Your skin in the treatment area may look as if it has been burnt by the sun. If your treatment is taking place during the summer don't allow this area to get any more sun. It is not recommended to wash this area with soap, just splash the effected part with luke warm water and gently dry without rubbing. You should not use lotions, hot water bottles, ice packs, or deodorants on the area either. If you are finding a problem with this mention it to the radiographer as they may have some cream which will help you.

Radiation after a TURP can apparently increase the risk of stricture (this is like a scar which on rehealing joins to adjacent tissue and causes a partial blockage), but this can be minimised if the radiotherapy treatment is delayed for two months after the TURP operation.

A study in the USA, reported in RAD magazine in January 1995, compared radiation therapy to radical prostatectomy. The results indicated that radiation therapy was comparable to a radical prostatectomy in controlling localised prostate cancer, i.e. cancer which was still confined to the prostate gland. Ten year survival rates for patients with the earliest stage of prostate cancer was 100% dropping to 40% for men with a cancer which had moved out of the prostate but had not invaded the lymph nodes or pelvic area. Other factors also showed radiation in a good light, in that incontinence, impotence and other complications all had lower incidences compared to surgery. On the financial side the cost was cheaper with outpatient treatment compared to hospitalisation for surgery.

There is some evidence that MAB **(maximum androgen blockade)** (see page 41) used before radiation treatment will increase its effectiveness. This is because the MAB reduces the number of cancer cells by up to 50% in some cases. This gives the radiotherapy a much better chance of destroying the remainder.

* **RADIOACTIVE IMPLANTS.** Radioactive pellets or 'seeds' implanted directly into the prostate gland can now be given, these irradiate the prostate and the surrounding tissue. The main advantage claimed for this method is that the dosage is concentrated close to the cancer and there is less harm done to adjacent tissue. The disadvantages so far noted are that if the seeds are not placed carefully then not all the cancer cells will be killed. There is also comment of a small risk of erosion of the rectal wall, and a possibility the seeds could move.

CHAPTER SEVEN

DRUG/HORMONE RELATED TREATMENT OPTIONS

As some 40% of patients when first seen have a prostate cancer which has moved out from the prostate capsule, removal of the prostate gland and radiotherapy is no longer an option. These patients would normally be recommended one of the following treatments. As up to 80% of prostate cancers 'initially' are hormone dependant, stopping the flow of testosterone reaching the prostate gland is the method used to stop/slow/reverse the progress of the cancer. Incidentally the world wide market for antiandrogen drugs was estimated at some £270 million in 1994.

* **ORCHIDECTOMY.** **(Surgical removal of the testes)**. Orchidectomy is regarded by the medical profession as a minor outpatient operation. The removal prevents the manufacture of testosterone by the testes. The testes manufacture approx. 95% of the body's testosterone. The remaining 5% is made by the adrenal gland. The results can be a reduction in the size of the tumour and a dramatic drop in any pain. Side effects include hot flushes, low sex drive, loss of muscle mass and impotence. Orchidectomy is also known to produce psychological problems. Even though the majority of testosterone is removed, testosterone and therefore DHT levels can still be as high as 40% of normal due to hormones from the adrenal gland. The cost of an orchidectomy is approx. £1,000 compared to £1,600 for a comparable drug treatment, see below. This operation is not the complete removal of the scrotal sack, just a portion of the interior.

* **HORMONES.** Can be a course of naturally occurring oestrogen's (hormones) such as ethinyl oestradiol or a man-made one such as stiboestrol. Oestrogens close down the

pituitary gland, which in turn would normally stimulate the testicles to make testosterone. Stiboestrol is the cheapest and, it has been reported, the most effective. There is comment that none of the LHRH treatments (see below) give better relief of symptoms or improved survival compared to stibestrol but they do avoid its side effects i.e. cardiovascular stroke, venous thrombosis, fluid retention and breast enlargement. Neither this course of oestrogen's nor orchidectomy stop the adrenal gland from making testosterone. The treatment needs to be taken for life. One urologist recently commented that stiboestrol should no longer be used as there are better treatments, (shown below), without the side effects linked to this hormone.

* **LHRH AGONISTS (Luteinzing Hormone Releasing Hormone)** (Gonadotropin releasing hormone analogues) (These consist of the drugs buserelin (Suprefact), goserelin (Zoladex) and leuprorelin (Prostap)), given as a monthly injection. Longer-lasting, three monthly injections are now available. The cost to the NHS of a single three month injection is £366. The testes and adrenal glands will only manufacture testosterone if they receive a hormone signal from a part of the brain, the pituitary gland. LHRH agonists act directly on the pituitary and prevent the signal from occurring. What they do is overstimulate the gland until it is exhausted.

The loss of testosterone produces side effects such as hot flushes, low sex drive, loss of muscle mass and impotence. Many men will also get a flare up of symptoms initially after treatment with an LHRH drug as the overstimulation of the pituitary which produces the 'signal' hormone creates an excessive output of the 'signal' hormone. The flare can cause enhanced pain and an enlargement of the tumour, there is also a chance of walking difficulties from any tumour growth in the spine area. This flare **must be** prevented by a preliminary treatment with cyproterone or flutamide. These two drugs stop the testosterone which is in the body reaching the prostate gland.

Some tumours are not effected by a loss of testosterone and in the longer term these treatments are not a permanent solution for cancers that initially react to testosterone loss and progress to a form which is resistant to hormone deprivation. The duration of response to hormonal therapy averages out at some 18 months, but much longer periods have been seen in individual patients.

In other words imagine there are two types of cancer, one type will grow with or without testosterone being present. The other needs testosterone to grow. Stop the testosterone and the second type of cancer will slow down, stop, or even shrink. The problem is that this second type of cancer will eventually change and will begin to grow again, even though its supply of testosterone is cut off.

* **ANTI-ANDROGENS**. Rather than stopping the production of testosterone these drugs, **cyproterone acetate and flutamide**, are anti-androgens and they block the effects of the testosterone, [after production], on the tumour. Another way of looking at it is that they bind to the prostate cells and prevent the ingress of testosterone, so the testes and adrenal manufacture away but the testosterone cannot reach the prostate gland because it is blocked by the action of these drugs. It is understood that many men will not become impotent if they take this treatment.

Not all the hormones which 'feed' the cancer are stopped by just one drug or treatment and this is where total androgen blockade comes in. Having said that, it is known that as many as 20-25% of prostate cancers are not affected by the withdrawal of hormones. Of greater concern is that many, which are sensitive, change and are no longer dependant upon hormones, whether formed in the testes or the adrenal gland.

* **MAB.   TOTAL OR MAXIMUM ANDROGEN BLOCKADE**. When a patient is given cyproterone or flutamide to stop a flare-up which is produced when a patient is given Zoladex, this dual treatment stops all possible chance of any testosterone getting to the prostate. This in effect is what is known as MAB. There is a school of thought that a permanent use of these two drug regimes (an anti-androgen & an LHRH) is the solution to prostate cancer at this stage. This is achieved, as noted previously, by stopping the signals which stimulate the adrenal gland and testes to produce testosterone and then backing that up with cyproterone or flutamide which stops any 'loose'

testosterone that may still be getting through from binding to the tumour. There is some evidence that this method of treatment prolongs life and helps the patient. As you might imagine this total blockade increases the overall cost. The average survival period for a man with metastatic cancer is two years, but with new treatments coming along this time could be extended.

As mentioned in chapter 13, MAB reduces the size of tumours. So MAB followed by radiotherapy for instance can be an effective treatment with a possiblity of a cure. Regrettably there is evidence that some GP'S are refusing MAB treatment to their patients. If this happens to you then **create. Remember that the medics job is to advise, it is yours to decide.** Do not be put off by an argument that the treatment is expensive and has bad side effects. Medics are using much more expensive drugs with far higher toxicity than these blockers, on other forms of cancers.

Here is an extract from the Medical Defence Union guidelines :-

" **.... in consenting to treatment every patient has the right to make his or her own decision regarding medical treatment and care, and in order to make that decision is entitled to have full information about the material risks. The clinicians duty is to supply the information in sufficient detail to enable the patient to make that decision.!"**

There is at least one drug which claims to blockade all on its own. Currently known as CB7630 it is still under development.

* **MARIMASTAT.** In December 1995 the largest UK biotech company, Oxford based British Biotec, announced the results of a clinical trial of some 91 patients. It was stated that over 50% had responded well to the treatment and 33% had either a reduction or a stabilisation in the size of the cancer. The side effects are described as modest and have been put down to the high dosage used in the trials, it is understood that 4% of the patients actually withdrew from the trials because of these side effects.

Marimastat appears to protect normal cells from being attacked by an adjacent cancer. What seems to happen is that the drug puts a shell around the cancer and cuts off its blood supply. This drug has been used not only for prostate cancer but also for cancer of the womb, the pancreas and the colon.

But be aware it is very much early days yet, only a very small trial has been carried out so far. A company spokesman has announced that a further two years of clinical tests, using lower doses, and regulatory paperwork lie ahead. A further 250 patients are currently in the second series of trials. One newspaper report stated that the drug cannot be made available to patients unless they are within a trial. So if you feel that this is the direction you want to travel ask your GP to see if he can get you on the next trial. Certainly you can expect expanding trials over the next 18 months as the company attempts to pass Phase III trials and seeks the approval of the US Food and Drug Administration. There is no indication yet that the drug 'cures'; note that only some 50% found some betterment and there is no advice about any longer term problems with the drug.

* **CHEMOTHERAPY.** Clinical trials on such products as Suramin are being carried out but with no satisfactory results to date. Suramin interferes with the surface receptors on the cell but there appears to be no evidence that any form of chemotherapy has shown any success in halting the progression of the disease or helped in the survival of a patient.

* **RESEARCH.** It is always possible that the hospital you are attending may be conducting a clinical trial of some new type of drug or method of dealing with prostate cancer. You should take great care before you make any decision in this regard. Ensure you have the fullest information. How would it alter the treatment you would normally have had for instance ? Try to discuss this with three or more people who are involved with the trial. You may find that different aspects of the 'trial' come out in later conversations which had not been apparent initially. No matter how well spoken, officious, or apparently superior the person is who is asking you to take part in a trial, he or she will not be offended if you say no, or that you would like to think about it. Remember you are not required to do this if you do not

wish to, it is simply a voluntary act on your part and will have no bearing on your future relationship with the specialist or the treatment you are going to receive.

* **LONG TERM COMPLICATIONS.** Very rarely surgical intervention might be required if the tumour obstructs the rectum. Surgical treatment may also be needed to prevent paraplegia if there is spinal cord compression.

CHAPTER EIGHT

PAIN TREATMENT & CARE.

Death is not the primary concern of a man with metastatic cancer, but pain control is. Metastatic cancer is cancer which has moved out from the prostate, to other parts of the body. Another term for such new cancers is secondaries.

Cancers have a known spread, for instance lung cancers can spread to the brain, breast and prostate cancers to the bone. If a prostate cancer has caused no urinary problems for the patient, or he has ignored the symptoms, then this spread away from the prostate into the lymphatic glands and bones and the subsequent pain is what will probably compel a man to visit his GP. The pain can be caused by several factors, from a localised site within the bone, to spinal cord or root compression. This can be associated with nerve problems which may require neurosurgical intervention.

Dispensing problems occur for both GP and patient. There is fear that the patient will become addicted to the drugs which are used for pain relief but this has been shown to be virtually never the case, and there is concern that narcotic drugs can give side effects such as nausea, vomiting, drowsiness and constipation. Finally there is also medical evidence that the drugs can be used to overdose, or cause cardiac arrest or respiratory problems.

So are there any medical guide lines for pain control ? Will your medical team prescribe what you want when you want, or are they bound by rules which will prevent you receiving the pain relief you need ? The answer is no, there are **no** guide lines. It is up to your medical team to ensure that you are pain free, so the more you confide in them the better they will be able to ensure that pain does not become a controlling part of your daily life.

Control is sometimes achieved by drugs, even aspirin, but mainly morphine, as this blocks off pain signals. It is far better to take a drug before the pain begins than it is to take it after pain has begun, the latter method means you will have to await the sedative effect to begin, the former means you will never be troubled at all. By the way, being prescribed morphine is not a sign that the medical team have written you off and they are about to wind you down (!), it is a sign that **you** want to pursue as full a life as possible in the circumstances, with full control of any pain that there maybe.

If you ever suffered from BPH (the non cancerous enlargement of the prostate gland), which meant you had to get up several times each night, you will know how this continued waking can exhaust you and mean that the next day you are 'good for nothing'. This is why you must, with your medical team, set up a good regime to enable you to always get a good nights sleep with no waking up with pain. Not all the pain a man will experience is directly from the cancer, it may be as a result of treatment to control the cancer.

Physical activity produces endorphins which can act as pain killers. The opposite, lack of activity depresses these endorphins so some sort of daily routine which helps in this regard would seem to be a good way of depressing the pain threshold.

But when other methods have failed radiotherapy can be a good option for bone metastases. This takes the form of half body radiation, relief appears within 48 hours but side effects such as nausea, vomiting, radiation pneumonia and bone marrow depression are all reported. (See page 36)

If at any time you are suffering pain which your medical team appear to be unable to get to grips with ask for a pain specialist, this would probably be an oncologist. Not only will he or she be knowledgeable about bone pain, which needs different treatments to other cancer induced pain, but the oncologist would also know of any new drugs which could help. Remember you are entitled to ask for and to receive such skilled advice. At the back of the book you will find the addresses of two Pain Centre help lines, if you require help or want to discuss your problems they are only a phone call away.

* METASTRON. In 1994 a new drug came on the market which is not a narcotic. Metastron is a radioactive (strontium-90) product which has had half a dozen clinical trials involving over 500 patients. Up to 50% of those taking part found they had excellent results with almost a complete loss of bone pain. The drug is injected intravenously and is taken up by the bone in the same way as calcium is absorbed. Although taken up by all bone it concentrates in the areas of the cancerous growth. It can stop bone pain completely and may even kill some cancerous cells. Pain reduction can take approx. two weeks to become apparent, but can last for over a full year, although the average time is six months, further injections can be given every 90 days. There is currently no limit to the number of injections which can be given.

The disadvantage of using Metastron is that patients will experience an increase, a flare up, of bone pain for possibly two days some 40 hours after the injection. You should ensure that you have something to hand to temper this effect. An oral narcotic would probably be suitable. The radioactivity of the drug can also cause a drop in the white blood cells and platelet counts for approx. one to two months after the initial injection. Usually things will revert to normal by the end of the third month. One clinical trial showed a reduced amount of analgesics required, a good improvement in the quality of life and a reduction of new metastases in patients using Metastron. A further study comparing half body radiotherapy with Metastron indicated that Metastron was as effective as the radiation.

Based on this trial it would seem that there are less apparent side effects with Metastron compared to radiation for a similar improvement of pain relief. Readers should note that there has been no **major** trial of most of the treatments mentioned. This means that some of the results may not always be borne out in practice.

All these treatments may be good for the body but do they help the inner man ? Can they enhance the spirit, rev up the energy motor when it starts to run down ? One way of doing that is by getting involved with a group.

Regrettably there is only one prostate cancer group at the moment. Men don't seem very good at 'grouping up'. It appears that meeting others with the same condition can not only help the 'patient' but also the rest of the family, as it allows them to talk freely, for they know that the others in the group all have similar problems. No one feels that they are pushing their personal baggage onto an outsider who has no conception of the problems of being a man with prostate cancer or the family who are caring for him. Meetings don't have to be formal. They can just be coffee and biscuits, one morning a month, or they can be formal with a nurse or GP present to answer questions and advise on the latest treatments and care in your local area. There is some suggestion that following such group meetings the participants immune system is considerably boosted and survival rates are higher compared to those who take the lone road. For those who prefer to write to someone with prostate cancer, then the PHA have a Support Network, (see the Useful addresses at the back of the book).

The most important person not mentioned so far is the carer. Sometimes the load they have to carry proves almost too great and this means that the care they are able to give will deteriorate. A clinical psychologist should be available at your local hospital, so ask for support. If your carer has been looking after you day and night for a long time they also may be suffering. So regardless of your feelings about having someone else to help out, and in spite of your carer saying that she can manage 'perfectly well thank you', there will come a time when it is sensible that some of the care is received from outside the home, if only to allow your carer to have an occasional day or two of respite, time alone to rest, gather themselves and recharge. At the back of this book are help organisations.

If your cancer is diagnosed as aggressive then one of the first people you want to get to know is a Macmillan nurse. You should be able to contact one via your GP or hospital, or there is a telephone number at the back of this book. Not only are they trained in all aspects of cancer but also in the trauma which effects the patient and family. So an early contact means that they may even be able to liase with your specialist to ensure that you understand all that is going on, and what is more important, are able to convey to the medical team any anxieties you have about your future.

Any possible nursing may involve your community nurse, but don't forget the support, of a Marie Curie nurse who can step in to help the carer.

There are lots of ways to skin the cat, a horrible phrase, but certainly there are a lot of ways to nurse, to help, to enhance a persons quality of life, the carer as well as the patient. So don't be shy to think of some of the alternative treatments which are available. Reflexology, massage of various kinds, acupuncture, hypnotherapy and psychotherapy may all help directly during treatments and also in pain control.

In practical ways you must also look at your financial position. Don't wait until your are on your uppers, by that time the added weight of money worries may drag you downward faster than the cancer you have. Use the addresses at the back of the book, if they cannot help they may know of an organisation who can. Your GP, nurse, CAB (Citizens Advice Bureau), all will have contacts which may lead to assistance. Maybe you can no longer drive but need to visit a treatment centre a good distance away. Ask, for all you know a local organisation already has such a service up and running. The words 'social workers' seem to be linked almost totally these days to abused children. Yet this is only one aspect of their work load and they are skilled, or should be, in assessing the needs of those who are in your position. So once again don't wait until your back is breaking. Get some advice.

BEWARE. One of the problems in this world is that there are crooks of many shades of gray. Some are only too willing to take advantage of anyone be they old or sick, you must count amongst them those who give the impression that they can cure your cancer and are willing to do so for inflated sums of money. It is in fact illegal to claim such things and because of that the claims made may be a little more subtle. But that should not stop you exploring the alternative therapies which may help you cope with day to day living. (See The Alternative View, Chapter 10). As with the medical profession, before you embark on such a course there is nothing wrong with obtaining a second opinion to ensure that the 'treatment' you are taking is valid and you are not becoming a victim.

One thing you will find, as with any long term project is that 6 months down the line you will be unable to remember accurately just what date you started this drug, or when you stopped the treatment etc. If you are sunk in gloom and despair this will not be of interest to you, but if you are alert and 'giving it a go' then such facts will be. So what would be of use will be a diary or note pad so that you can enter events as they happen. Knowing that visits from the grandchildren mean that the next day you have more pain than normal may only be revealed in a day to day account, and will allow you to compensate by taking things a little easier for instance. There are many things which will prevent you from having a good quality of life. If you are able to distinguish what these are then you can cut them out or work around the problem to eliminate it.

CHAPTER NINE

PREVENTION ?

Can prostate cancer be avoided ? There is so much that is not known about prostate cancer that the answer to that question is wide open. However, from what is known and from what has been written and is currently going on in the prostate world, several logical conclusions can be drawn. Acting on them may not make any difference. Current studies being published may lead to nothing, so you must read as much as you can then come to your own decision.

In much of the literature about prostate cancer time and time again, the message comes through that prostate problems are hormone related.

* Prostate cancer is treated by depriving the cancer of testosterone, either by surgical or drug castration, which means it cannot be changed to DHT, which in turn allows the cancer to grow.

* PIN (see page 67) an apparent precursor of prostate cancer [by some ten years] is decreased when the body is given androgen blockading drugs.

Merck Pharmaceuticals are testing their drug Proscar on some 18,000 men in a long term study to see if it affects the rate of prostate cancer deaths. (Proscar is a drug which prevents the conversion of testosterone into DHT (dihydro-testosterone)). This trial, which will last some 7 years, began late in 1993. It is obvious that someone at this Pharmaceutical company believes that reducing the levels of DHT could have an effect. So much so that they are willing to allocate a considerable sum of money to test it.

* The growth of BPH is dependent on the steroid 5 alpha reductase converting testosterone into DHT. Stop the **steroid** working in this way and the theory is you stop the growth. PROSCAR has been shown to reduce the levels of DHT in the blood by an average of 65%..

Testosterone reduces in the male as he gets older, so it appears strange that his chances of contracting prostate cancer increases the older he gets, the converse would be the obvious conclusion. However if the PIN, and hence the prostate cancer, are 'triggered' early in a mans life by testosterone (DHT), then the natural lowering of his testosterone levels by old age come in much too late to be of any help.

What evidence is there that abnormal prostate growth can be triggered early in life ? Well the reader has to travel across to the American continent to a small village in the Dominican Republic. Back in the 1970's researchers found children in this village who were raised as females until they reached the age of 12, at this point they put on body-weight and in effect turned into boys. When born they had female sexual organs, but at 12 they developed a functional penis. Locally these children are known as GUEVEDOCES (penis at age 12). As they mature they develop a tiny prostate, their hairline does not recede and they never get acne.

These events published in an American magazine set in motion the research and development of the drug PROSCAR. It was shown that there was a common genetic deficiency which caused males to be born with what is best described as ambiguous external parts. The deficiency is in **steroid** 5 alpha reductase. Researchers used this shortage to identify which androgen is responsible for what effect in male development.

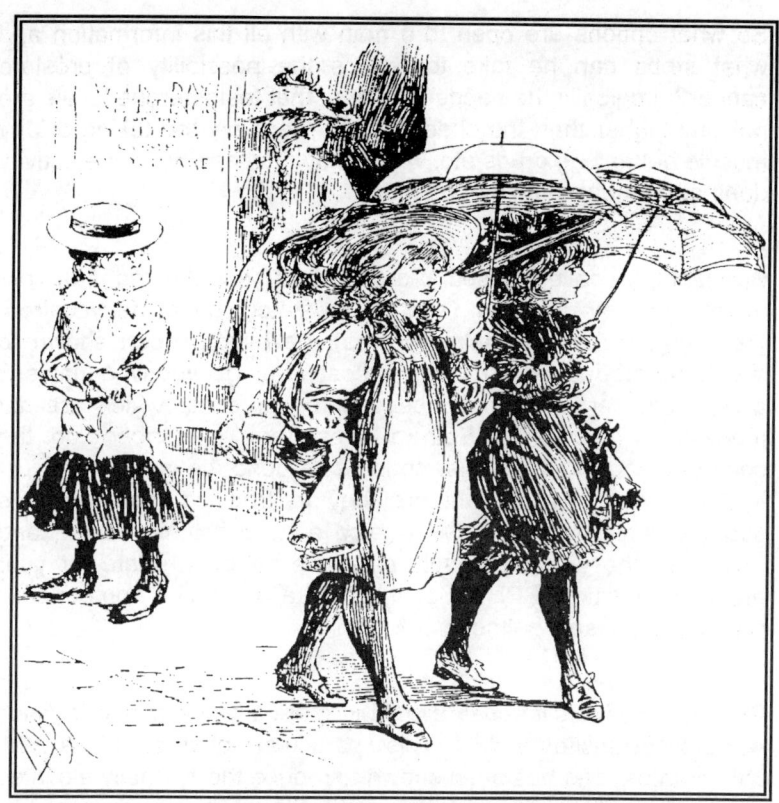

"...... raised as females until they reached the age of twelve"

The lack of DHT in the bodies of the children inhibited the growth of the prostate. It also apparently turns out that these children never have a prostate enlargement as they reach old age, [no comment is made as to prostate cancer]. So does the action of DHT prior to age twelve 'switch' the prostate cells on to produce an enlarged benign growth ? Only further research will tell.

To summarize:- your body produces testosterone which converts to DHT and causes benign enlargement. It also helps in the growth of a prostate cancer. Stop the DHT conversion and you stop the benign enlargement. **What is not known is:- will early use of a DHT inhibitor stop prostate cancer ?**

So what options are open to a man with all this information and what steps can he take to reduce the possibility of prostate cancer? Logically, he needs to ensure that testosterone levels are not any higher than they need to be. Certainly the taking of any muscle enhancing drugs etc. which may increase hormone activity does not appear to be a good idea.

Prostabrit, a pollen based prostate treatment derived from rye grass and saw palmetto, (another prostate product derived from the berry of the saw palmetto tree), have both been shown to inhibit the production of DHT. To those amongst you who may shy away from herbal or 'over the counter' products which are not medically prescribed. Both of these are 'prescribed' on the continent and in many other countries around the world. It is just in the UK that, in some quarters, they are frowned upon, which is strange because if your GP is also a homeopathic doctor, and many are, he would probably prescribe sabel serrulata for your prostate condition (BPH). Sabel serrulata is in fact a homeopathic preparation of saw palmetto.

From clinical trials it appears that there are a range of plants which contain Beta-sitosterol. This particular phytosterol is anti inflammatory and has been shown to reduce the normally elevated levels of prosaglandins in patients with BPH. The rye grass pollen extract which forms the basis of Prostabrit and the saw palmetto berry extracts, such as Prostex, which form the basis of several 'over the counter' prostate preparations are two preparations which contain B-sitosterol. The Lancet, in June 1995, reported a clinical trial on B-sitosterol, which indicated a significant improvement in symptoms and in urinary flow for men with BPH, although they added that it was unlikely that there was any **substantial** effect on the size of the prostate. As the trial was only for a period of six months perhaps a longer period would have a more positive effect. Going back to the previous sentence just what do they mean by substantial ? If they feel a substantial effect (reduction in size) on the size of the gland would be 75%, and this 'was unlikely' does that mean that there could have been an effective reduction of 50% ? It seems unlikely that the subject would have been mentioned at all unless there had been some effect on the prostate size. But we will probably never know.

Is it possible that the inclusion of b-sitosterol in the diet for a decade or two would be of help ? Would it stop the prostate being washed with large amounts of DHT for 10 or 20 years prior to the age of 60 if a man took such DHT inhibitors, but more importantly would it stop or lower the incidence of benign and malignant growth ?.

An alternative, if you don't want to take tablets or capsules is to increase the amount of fibre in your diet. Beans, peas, lentils and many dried fruits etc. allow a greater binding to hormones like testosterone which reduce the amount in the body.

Digression..

If the market for anti androgen drugs is worth £270 million and you add on to that all the other few hundred millions that the pharmaceutical companies get for drug related treatments for prostate cancer and BPH treatments, that's a lot of cash !. If B-sitosterol actually could stop/reduce the incidence, not only of BPH but also prostate cancer, would **they** ever let it become public knowledge ? (Of course they would).

But back to the issue in hand.......

IS FOOD THE ANSWER ?.

The medical world have attempted to link diet directly to the human prostate cancer and have failed with the exception of a link with saturated fat. Nevertheless, as it is a fact that a man from the Far East has a low percentage chance of prostate cancer until he moves to the West, then food could be one of the factors which will increase his risk. Asian men eat more green vegetables and a minimum of meat. Much of this diet, not normally adopted by Western man, such as soya based foods, grains, tofu, contain substances that the body converts into weak oestrogen 'type' hormones. These oestrogens are also found in some of the more unusual members of the cabbage family such as Chinese leaves and Kohlrabi. The theory is that these combine/react with the body's own hormones and in some way protect against BPH (there is no direct evidence they influence cancer). Blood levels of dietary oestrogens are 100 times higher in Asian races compared to Western man.

There is a report that environmental oestrogens from sources such as dioxins, traces of female HRT and oral contraceptive pills in drinking water are currently implicated in the increased incidence of prostate cancer.

If that is so how can one lot of oestrogens be thought to prove beneficial whilst others are harmful ? It appears that plant oestrogens are sufficiently similar to those in the human body in that they trigger the production of a protein which gathers up dietary oestrogens as well as male hormones and deactivates them. In this way the prostate has a reduced exposure to hormones. Synthetic environmental oestrogens are not subdued in this way as they do not trigger the production of the protein. So it would seem prudent to **cut out red meat and animal fat and to increase the amount of fruit and green and yellow leafed vegetables and soya based foods in your diet**.

Before we leave hormones, synthetic or otherwise, I note that caffeine is alleged to stimulate the adrenal gland. I have not seen that it actually stimulates it to release more testosterone but as caffeine-free tea and coffee are easily obtainable it would seem sensible to switch. Some meat and dairy products are also known to contain hormones which have been used to increase milk yield or to promote growth, possibly another area to avoid or at least cut down to a minimum input.

Researchers in the USA followed up 51,000 men who completed periodic food frequency questionnaires. In 300 cases of prostate cancer, animal fat, especially from red meat seemed to increase the risk of prostate cancer by just over 60%.

Recent work by Dr. Yu Wang and some colleagues in New York have shown that a low fat diet can slow or reverse the growth of prostate cancer in animals. So once again a fat intake has been shown to be related to prostate cancer risk. **So a low animal fat, high fibre diet appears to be a must**. Even the BMJ in 1994 published research results on vegetarian diets which supported the view that low protein diets lessened the chances of cancer. (This was not a survey on prostate cancer).

Comment in regard to Asian men having a lower chance of prostate problems, and the reason appearing to be a diet low in animal fat and high in soya, coincides with a Lancet report in 1993. This stated that soya is a rich source of isoflavanoids which inhibit the growth of prostate cancer. **So soya products would also appear to assist a man who wishes to prevent prostate problems.**

You may have seen much in the press over the last few years about 'free radicals' and 'antioxidants'. Apparently the cells of the body have some 100,000 free radicals colliding with them every day. To put it as simply as possible, this can produce damage to the DNA. Imagine that every time a cell in the body has to be repaired or reproduced, a reference has to be made to the DNA master plan, if the plan has been damaged the new cell may be lacking an essential component. This may be the reason for a cell to go out of control, if that cell is a prostate cell the reasoning is that it could initiate a prostate cancer.

Eating a diet rich in antioxidant vitamins and minerals can reduce the amount of free radicals in the body. (Cut down the chance of the DNA getting damaged). Yes, you have guessed it, Asians eat many more of the foods which contain these vitamins, peppers, broccoli, and spinach for instance. You will also find capsules for sale in your Health food store or check with your Pharmacist. What you need to look out for are Vitamin C, beta carotene, zinc and selenium, all of these are regarded as anti-oxidant vitamins and minerals.

It has been shown that a healthy prostate has high levels of zinc. A report in 'What Doctors Don't Tell You', stated, " Compared with other groups, men with the most malignant form of prostate cancer have the highest cadmium levels and the lowest zinc levels. Studies have shown that zinc supplements can successfully reduce an enlarged prostate and treat the associated symptoms. **It is therefore suggested that a daily 15 mg. dose of zinc forms part of our diet.....**" Zinc rich foods consist of whole grains, seafoods, nuts, eggs, to name a few.

Essential fatty acids such as linseed and sunflower seeds are thought to reduce the risk of prostate cancer cells forming.

Keeping out of the sun to avoid cancer is now the watch word, but is it being overplayed ? Another survey from the U.S. indicates that vitamin D, made by the body after exposure to sunlight, may be playing a role in reducing the risk of prostate cancer. So a moderate amount of sunlight, or taking more Vit D could be helpful. A recent report in the Lancet showed that the levels of vitamin D in over a third of men over 60 was below normal range. Apparently the daily recommended dose of vitamin D for a 60+ year old is up to 800 units, more than we can get from the average diet.

Earlier this century, an American called Edgar Cayce regularly went into a 'trance state' and diagnosed thousands of medical problems and suggested treatments. His efforts are well documented and there is now a world wide Cayce movement, very active here in the UK. In one reading for someone who wanted a 'treatment' which would help avoid cancer, Cayce said simply "eat three almonds a day".

So eat three almonds a day.

Scientists are carrying out a survey in a further attempt to link diet and prostate cancer. This study, code named EPIC, is due to run for 10 years. (Nothing is quick in the world of prostate cancer). 400,000 men are being checked across nine countries, this includes some 40,000 men in the UK. The volunteers, as well as recording everything they eat, will also give annual blood and urine samples. The hope is that as individual volunteers develop cancer the scientists will be able to find some common cause in the records they have accumulated.

One last mention of Asian diets. Male baldness is androngen dependent. Hair loss is thought to be related to the DHT in the hair root. Not only do Asian men have a lower susceptibility to prostate problems they are also less prone to baldness. So although in general male body hair is dependent upon testosterone, hair on the male head is in fact decreased by the subsequent breakdown to DHT. This leads to the thought that not only could you be lowering your chances of prostate problems if you make a change of diet you could also be improving your chances of keeping your crowning glory for a much longer period of time ! All in all the Asians seem to be a lucky race !

CHAPTER TEN

THE ALTERNATIVE VIEW

Whatever you may think of the word alternative it is only alternative depending upon where you stand. Martin J. Walker writing in WDDTY in June 1995 wrote, "up until the end of the second world war, great strides had been made in identifying vitamins and minerals and relating these elements to human health and nutrition. Dr Max Gerson treated cancer with 'cleansing' diets based on fruit and vegetables. Dr Max Birchner-Benner cured patients of a variety of illnesses with a regime based on raw fruits and vegetables. But by the mid 60's, old ideas about wholefoods and the high quality nutritional status of vegetables and fruits changed". So now-a-days such ideas are not in the mainstream of medical practice.

THE GERSON DIET. This diet is still in use. The time expended on this treatment is immense, one man who is trying it appears to have little time for anything else but the regime. To ensure the body is clean of toxins the following 'foods' are out:- Sugar, fats, alcohol, tea, coffee, salt, tobacco and any food that contains preservatives or additives.

Amongst the foods you can eat are vegetables which should be organically grown. Vegetables may be steamed but raw vegetables are recommended. Seeds which are rich in protein such as pulses (peas, lentils, beans), pumpkin and sunflower, apricot kernels, sesame and nuts. Fresh fruit or dried is aok.

The main part of the regime is that you should be taking some 2 pints per day of liquidized vegetables and fruit. It is recommended that you obtain full detail from someone local who is in a position to supervise your treatment. Check out the local alternative health centre. It is recommended you only drink spring or mineral water.

* **THE BRISTOL DIET.** This was a strict diet similar to a Gerson diet, although it appears to have been modified somewhat in recent years. More detail of this from the books produced by the Bristol Cancer Help Centre.

* **MACROBIOTIC DIET** The macrobiotic diet has a history going back decades. Although this is mainly a vegan diet and consists of large amounts of raw vegetables with half of each meal meant to consist of wholewheat cereals, it is supposed to be 'prescribed' for each person by a teacher. Although it prohibits many of the items mentioned in the Gerson diet it varies from it considerably. So if you are keen you need to read up on the subject and find yourself a guide, (see the useful addresses at the back of the book).

Your medical adviser will, in all probability, not recommend and will not be happy if you try these diets. One conventional medical advice comment stated "these diets are low in energy, high in fibre and difficult to follow". An alternate way would be to cut out meat and try a vegetarian diet

* **VITAMINS.** There is strong support for the idea that cancer is a sign of lack of vitamins and that mega doses can help. Vitamin C appears to have a good reputation vis a vis cancer. Comment varies from cancer patients surviving four times longer than expected when taking vitamin C, to a superior effectiveness of conventional treatments when taken in conjunction with the vitamin. As Vitamin C is alleged to enhance immunity and neutralise toxins it makes sense. As the whole point is that you take mega amounts of the vitamin, once again you need to obtain guidance before you embark on this course. (See Useful address)

* **POSITIVE THINKING.** It wasn't long ago that if you had a serious illness then only medical treatment would help and everything else was superfluous. Yet now more and more positive thinking is becoming an acceptable part of medical treatment. "Day by Day in every way I am getting better and better", is an old repetitive phrase which is supposed to improve your whole outlook on life and change your world forever. Now

adays it is a little more structured with a touch of the meditations and some visualization thrown in.

Professor Bob Lewin of Hull University, believes that positive thinking is vital for his patients. He has devised a rehabilitation programme which is in use in 80 NHS hospitals. He quotes the situation of 14 angina patients who improved to such an extent under his program that they no longer required heart surgery.

Another professor, Karol Sikora, also backs up Professor Lewins ideas. He advises that he has had patients with secondary bone cancers who have survived for 20 years. He knows that people who have survived for longer than expected tend to make light of their condition. **Although it is no guarantee it appears to be helpful to be positive about your condition**.

All this positive thinking needs a structure and physical fitness programmes, with input from yoga. One of the things which is well known is that athletes who train hard get a 'fix' from the endorphins which are released by the body. These are in fact our own personal morphine injections and they give a personal high. What better way to help yourself through the trauma of prostate cancer than to take advantage of your own ability to release these endorphins which are also known to lift depression. Regular exercise can do just that. It is understood that just a 2 mile walk can be enough to trigger such action. Exercise is also thought to improve the immune system by increasing the number of white blood cells.

A PHA Subscriber advised that a serious effort on his part to increase his exercise regime before his radiotherapy treatment started, made a big difference to his treatment, in that he had virtually no side effects and he considered that it helped alot toward the success of the treatment.

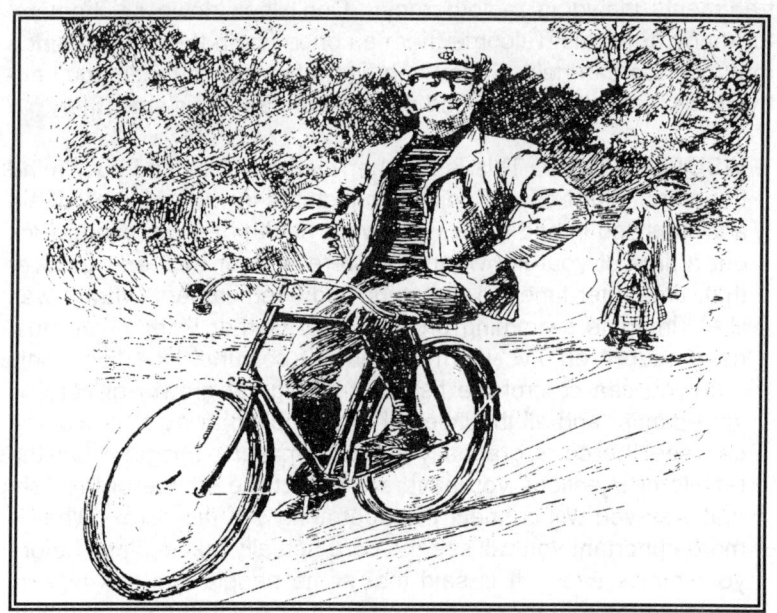

"The body has the ability to release endorphins. Regular exercise can trigger such action"

This is not violent exercise we are talking about but walking, cycling, or swimming.

At some time in the past you must have been in a room full of an 'electrical field' of tension. It may have been caused by emotional stress between the people in the room but whatever, it illustrates that people can radiate such tension.

If you are in a state of tension you will not only affect yourself but also those around you. There is comment that such tension within a body can stop all self healing; it certainly does not make for a good relationship between you and your partner, so try to relax this tension away for your own sake.

None of these suggestions have any clinical support that they will cure a cancer, but there is much evidence that it can enhance the quality of life in many respects. Hypnosis together with other techniques are known to reduce the side effects of many treatments including radiotherapy. Don't look down on 'healers' for many hospitals welcome them as once again there is evidence that they too can help. If you can find a teacher to teach you self-hypnosis you will certainly find the road ahead much smoother.

* **VISUALIZATION.** This is another method of getting your mind to control your body. Conjure up pictures in your mind of all the activities you intend to do when your health has improved. Pick out a time of your life when you were at your best and go over that, time after time, so that your body 'remembers' what it was like. Imagine swimming on the Great Barrier Reef, you must have seen it on TV, with hundreds of colourful little fish, only now you can control the fish and that great growth of coral is your cancer and all the little fish are nibbling away at it and you can see the coral gradually getting smaller. Imagine that the tablets or injections you have are in fact the source of the fish, that way you will connect the treatment with the cure. What is more important you will see the cure actually taking place before your minds eye. It is said that some people find this type of visualization too aggressive and by way of contrast one patient imagined her body as a garden and as she went around it she weeded out the 'cancer weeds' and offered the flowers she wanted to keep, care, compost and fertiliser. Constant repetition of such visualization techniques are reputed to reap rich rewards.

If you used the last technique you must complete it by looking at the picture of the garden and seeing it entirely weed free, all you will see is a perfect garden with not one blemish. Only in this way will your mind be able to implement the orders you are giving it to clear out the cancer cells totally.

Some research has been done in regard to improving the immune system, this is our own personal defence screen which will normally detect any cell in our body which is not required and kill it off. A tip top immune system can be achieved by a good diet and as noted,exercise. You will also find capsules in your health food shop that claim to help the immune system.

There is a school of thought that stress plays a part in cancer development. Stress can be brought on by work, or tension at home for instance. Being told you have prostate cancer can increase your stress levels and it is not helped by any apparent lack of concern by medical staff. This is where the alternative therapies can come in and one of the main ways to reduce stress appears to be yoga. You will find an address to help in this regard.

CHAPTER ELEVEN

STILL UNSURE ?

The side effects of some of these treatments (hormonal, surgery and radiotherapy) can shatter your self confidence if it hadn't already been shattered by the original diagnosis. Don't give up if you find you have problems, your GP should be able to help or refer you to someone who can. Impotence for instance can be managed by injections of caverject (alprostidil) or papaverine, or by the use of a vacuum pump.

As you can imagine there are many factors which need to be taken into account before any treatment is given. There is no standardized procedure which swings into force after a man is diagnosed with prostate cancer. Indeed there is much argument in the medical world about the type of treatment which should be given, this applies not only in the UK but around the world.

The results of the tests, the degree of advancement of the cancer, the health and age of the patient should all be taken into account. For instance do you give a man in his late 80's or 90's aggressive treatment such as surgery, radiotherapy and drugs, all of which can have violent effects on his current life style and which may never prolong his life at all, but will most certainly drastically reduce the quality of the years he has left? Or do you ensure that the remainder of his life span is made as comfortable as possible?

On the other hand the situation of a man in his 40's or 50's with family responsibilities could be viewed differently. It could be calculated that aggressive treatment would prolong his life and suppress the cancer for four or five years. The difficulty arises as you move the hypothetical patient's age down from the late 80's and up from the 50's. At what age do you decide treatment or comfort? An ethical dilemma.

To illustrate the benefits of 'watchful waiting' over actual treatments note the possible complications following the removal of the prostate, these apply whichever method is used. First there is a mortality risk because of the anaesthetic and the fact that the patient is having a major surgical operation. Then there are the possibilities of loss of bladder control (incontinence), infertility & impotence.

You may eventually have to make a choice from the treatments mentioned in this book. Put yourself in the driving seat today, so that if at some time in the future such a situation occurs, you are capable of taking the decision. Knowledge will give you the choice of controlling your life for as long as you wish to. This is just one collection of facts, your library will have books which can expand on what is written here.

One study of 95 patients, which was considered not large enough to be very accurate, showed that comparing radical prostatectomy, carried out immediately after diagnosis, to 'watch and wait' with treatment as and when needed (it did not say what that treatment was) produced no significant difference in survival. So in that case those who had the trauma of prostatectomy fared no better than those who avoided it.

Also with a bearing on this subject is a US Medicare survey on patients who had a radical prostatectomy in the period 1988-1990, 63% reported a day-to-day problem with a degree of incontinence, and 90% reported no erections sufficient for intercourse during the month prior to the survey. A statement in the survey was that preservation of potency is dependent upon tumour stage and patient age only. It makes no comment that it might also depend upon the expertise of the surgeon. Twenty-eight percent of these men also reported follow-up treatment for cancer with radiation or hormonal therapy within four years after the prostatectomy.

CHAPTER TWELVE

OTHER TYPES OF PROSTATE TUMOURS.

There are several other types of prostate cancer. Two of them, transitional cell and mixed ductal tumours are aggressive cancers and require the complete removal of both the prostate and the bladder assuming they are found whilst still confined to the prostate.

Another tumour type that may require the removal of both the bladder and the prostate are endometroid tumours. They are similar to some types of female uterine cancers. Radiotherapy can help with advanced cases as can hormonal treatment or in some cases chemotherapy.

Intraductal adenocarcinomas are treated initially by a radical prostatectomy. Whilst the final four on the list, carcinosarcomas, rhabdomysocarcomas, chondrosarcomas and osteosarcomas will probably require the removal of the prostate, bladder and adjacent pelvic structures. So far radiation, hormones, and chemotherapy are not effective.

A NEW THEORY ON PROSTATE CANCER.

* PIN **Prostatic Intraepithelial Neoplasia**. PIN to a layman can best be described as cancerous cells which are non-invasive and non-destructive.

Studies in the USA have indicated that PIN appears to predate the onset of prostate cancer by some ten years. Although PIN can be found in prostates without cancer present there is more in prostates when prostate cancer is present. Studies have shown a close relationship between PIN and cancer. Some PIN show genetic abnormalities similar in form to prostate cancer. Such irregularities help towards uncontrolled cell growth by effecting the chromosomes in the cancer cells.

The early appearance of PIN, up to ten years prior to prostate cancer, should lead to a better understanding of prostate cancer. It should also make for earlier diagnosis, and possible intervention. This is because there is a strong possibility that PIN can be affected by androgen blockade. This could mean that PIN is hormone dependent.

CHAPTER THIRTEEN

PARAGRAPHS TO PONDER.

Patients of advanced age or with serious medical problems should be seriously considered for observation with no active treatment. This is especially so with men who have low grade tumours. There have been no clinical studies to see if radical prostatectomy, radiation, or watchful waiting had any advantage in prolonging life in men with prostate cancer. When you consider the trauma that men who have treatments may have, this would appear to be an important aspect to look into for any man in this category.

IT'S ALL DONE WITH MIRRORS.

To give readers some degree of insight into the world of medicine as it relates to the prostate condition here are some comments from a US document : -

Radical prostatectomy followed by immediate orchidectomy is under clinical evaluation.

Systemic chemotherapy for hormone refractory disease is under clinical evaluation.

Antiandrogens as monotherapy or other hormonal therapies are under clinical evaluation.

In other words the medics are saying, we have a lot of possible treatments which may or may not do a good job, but we have no long term studies to confirm if what we **are** using is what we **should** be using.

Don W. W. Newling from the Netherlands relates this story about a patient who at the age of 52 had a prostate tumour. His PSA level was 65 ng/ml and there was no sign of spread to the bone. Not wanting surgery he was given Zoladex and flutamide, (blockade). His PSA level dropped and a test some four months later found no increased problems. A check was made to see if the tumour had reduced and as there were no problems with the lymph nodes he had a radical prostatectomy. No sign of tumour was found.

The reduction of tumour size by the use of these two drugs is now well established. So it might be worth considering if you are told that things have gone too far for a prostatectomy, because of the size of the tumour, that the use of these drugs, in this way, could reduce the size of the tumour and prostate to a size which would allow such an operation. This reduction will also reduce the risk of dissemination as well. A tumour is staged, [graded according to its size and of its aggressiveness]. The medical team will treat you based on that staging. But staging can be inaccurate. So once again the use of these drugs can open up a doorway to a successful treatment by 'downstaging', the tumour.

Another report on a number of patients noted that MAB (maximum androgen blockade) reduced prostate size by up to 50% after three months. 13 of the 40 patients had downstaging after the treatment, i.e. their tumour had reversed. One patient actually had no detectable tumour, like the Dutch patient above. The follow-up surgery was much easier and produced shorter surgery time and reduced blood loss. Of more interest to a patient however is that full continence was achieved immediately after the removal of the catheter by a greater proportion of those men who had had MAB.

No large scale trial has been reported as at publication date.

TAKING CHARGE

This is your battle, but there is no reason you have to face it alone. The medical profession can diagnose and give opinions. The information comes to you **for you to make a decision**. You **do not** have decisions made for you, take **charge** of the situation.

So double check the diagnosis.

Use the latest techniques to ensure that the biopsy is fully checked out.

Ask for a DNA analysis.

Check out the treatments, not forgetting the varied side effects.

Be prepared for some unpleasant possibilities, but do not lose heart.

Check out help groups and fellow sufferers who can exchange experiences and offer other support.

Ensure that you have the best advisors, if that means changing then change.

Tell everyone, you'll be surprised at the help you will receive from unexpected quarters.

Put in the forefront of your mind that of 83% men diagnosed as having prostate cancer only 17% will actually die from the disease.

Above all accept that you have evolved since birth through difficult stages to the person you are today. You look back and know that if you could live those periods again, with your current knowledge, you would make a better job of them. Take this on board, what it is telling you is that with knowledge you are better able to control life. These life changes will continue whilst you continue to live so accept this and assimilate all you can about prostate cancer, ensure that 10 years from now you will not say "if only................"

Use foresight now and not hindsight later.

The founder of the American support group for prostate cancer survivors says. "**... understanding the risk and benefits of treatment options and being involved in decisions are so important, because they erase fear.**"

LATE NEWS.

Authors late comment.

When I thought through the ideas in the chapter titled 'PREVENTION ?' I had seen no other comment on it. Previous hints at the use of Proscar, saw palmetto, and Prostabrit in the PHA Newsletters had provoked no comment from anyone neither lay persons nor medics. But I felt that it was worth including in the book.

Just prior to sending the text off to the printers what appears in my post, much to my surprise, (thanks to the sender), but an article in 'Alternative Therapies' for September 1995, an American publication. The article advises that the County Hospital in Seattle would by January 1996 establish a natural medicine clinic within the hospital.

Much of the discussion prior to the agreement on establishing the clinic occurred at the King County Council in Washington State and revolved around the benefits of treating prostate cancer with diet & natural medicines, comment was made on the lack of carotenes, (vitamin A), zinc, too much dietary fat, lack of fish and vegetable oils, lack of soy foods, and the inclusion of saw palmetto to alter the action of testosterone.

As with many things, be it supermarkets or out of town shopping malls, give it another ten or twenty years and we will also find such treatments here in the UK given by the GP and urologist. But do we have to wait that long ? Only by a groundswell of patients demanding such treatments from the medics, or if they are not available going and seeking them out from alternative sources will a change occur sooner.

An American urologist recently said on a US tv programme, "it is going to take us 10 or 15 years to check out all the current 'treatments' to see if any of them actually give a longer life span than not carrying out the treatment at all". That means that before the medical establishment can give any guarantees I will be in my seventies, (well I hope I will !) Or more likely many of us will be dead.

Whilst that urologists' comment is in regard to treatments and not preventative measures, there are currently no preventative methods being put forward by the medical profession, that means that men now in their 40's may have missed an opportunity to alter their dietary habits through lack of knowledge or uncertainty due to the lack of backup from the very medical authorities who currently admit to not having an answer to the prostate condition.

If the current medical establishment had a preventative, or guaranteed cure for prostate cancer or BPH then I would be the first to endorse it. But this is not so. So as none of these natural methods appear to harm and certainly follow through as a logical answer to the problem, it would seem sensible to open the gate and walk down the road until a better route is available.

APPENDIX

As covered in chapter five do not make any immediate decisions. Go home, discuss the situation with your family. If you are not clear on anything you need to go back to your GP or specialist and ask questions to ensure that you are 100% certain in all respects about your condition. If you have one, take along a small tape recorder, this will ensure you get every word 100% correct. If not then take a pad and pen. Make sure you write down all the information you need. Your GP would rather you did that than need a further visit in 24 hours because you have forgotten all that was said.

Don't expect your GP to answer all your queries without some questions from you, he may not have seen anyone with prostate cancer for some time and will not know what individual fears you have. Be prepared to ask about every aspect of your condition that you can think of. If you are already in pain from your condition you are not being a 'hard man' or 'brave' by denying it. Early pain control can mean that you can carry on as normal, still enjoy your daily life and even be 'nice' to your family. There is nothing like pain to break up a happy family.

These are the types of questions you need answers to from your GP or specialist..

What sort of cancer and is it still contained within the prostate ?
What type of treatment do you recommend ?
What side effects can I expect from this treatment ?
How would you help me overcome these side effects ?
In your opinion what will be the result of this treatment ?
What is my life expectancy with and without these treatments ?

What alternative treatment is available ?

What side effects can I expect from this alternative treatment ?

How would you help me overcome these side effects ?

In your opinion what will be the result of this treatment ?

What is my life expectancy with and without these treatments ?

Will any further treatment be required at a later date ?

If so, what will that be, what would be the side effects etc. ?

How often would I be required to attend hospital for check-ups ?

Will I be able to get back to work/normal activities ?

It is at this stage that you should say. "I would very much like a second opinion before I begin any treatment."

It is possible that the specialist you are talking to is a surgeon without a lot of experience of prostate cancer. There may well be a urologist or even another surgeon in your area who has a vast experience of your condition. Your current specialist will fully understand your concern. If for some reason this is not the case then you must contact your GP and let him know the situation.

This would also be a good time to contact BACUP and TENOVUS and discuss your condition with one of the trained nurses on the phone. You may know someone who has prostate cancer, talk to them, this will allow you to discuss each others concerns. If you do not know anyone, but would like to, the PHA have a Support Network which includes men with prostate cancer who are willing to correspond and will answer your letters.

Space to write down additional questions while you remember them.

HELPFUL ADDRESSES.

Most of these organisations are charities, this usually means that cash is tight. So if you write, at least send a couple of stamps for your reply.

THE ASSOCIATION FOR NEW APPROACHES TO CANCER,
5 LARKSFIELD,
ENGLEFIELD GREEN,
EGHAM,
SURREY, TW20 0RB.
TELEPHONE : 01784 433 610

This charity acts as a nerve centre for a network of cancer self help groups, therapists, yoga classes, alternative therapies, etc etc. Large sae please.

~~~

BACUP,
121/123 CHARTERHOUSE STREET,
LONDON, EC1M 6AA.
TELEPHONE : Cancer information service   0171 608 1611
　　　　　　　　Freephone　　　　　　　　　　0800 181 199

Experienced nurses answer telephones or written queries on every facet of cancer. Counselling, books and information sheets are available free to patients and their families.

~~~

BRISTOL CANCER HELP CENTRE,
GROVE HOUSE,
CORNWALLIS GROVE,
BRISTOL, BS8 4PG.
TELEPHONE : 01272 743 216

They have day and weekly residential courses for patients and families. The courses consist of counselling, visualization, meditation, dietary advice and much more.

~~~

BRITANNIA HEALTH PRODUCTS LTD.
GREATNESS LANE,
SEVENOAKS,
KENT, TN14 5BQ.
TELEPHONE : 01737 773304

Britannia distribute the rye grass pollen based Prostabrit in the UK. This is a prescription product in many countries, but not in the UK, for BPH and prostatitis, it is not sold or recommended in any way by the distributers for the treatment of prostate cancer. The reason it is mentioned here is because it contains Beta-sitosterol.

~~~

BRITISH ACUPUNCTURE ASSOCIATION,
34 ALDERNEY STREET,
LONDON, SW1V 4EU.
TELEPHONE : 0171 834 1012.

~~~

BRITISH ASSOCIATION FOR COUNSELLING,
1 REGENT PLACE,
RUGBY, CV1 2PJ.
TELEPHONE : 01788 578 328

BRITISH ASSOCIATION FOR SEXUAL AND MARITAL THERAPY,
PO BOX 63,
SHEFFIELD, S10 3TS.
Clinics who offer help for such problems.

BRITISH HERBAL MEDICINE ASSOCIATION,
FIELD HOUSE,
LYEHOLE LANE,
REDHILL,
BRISTOL, BS18 7TB.
TELEPHONE : 01934 862 994

BRITISH HOMEOPATHIC ASSOCIATION,
27A DEVONSHIRE STREET,
LONDON, W1N 1RJ.
TELEPHONE : 0171935 2163

BRITISH WHEEL OF YOGA,
1 HAMILTON PLACE,
BOSTON ROAD,
SLEAFORD, NG34 7ES.
TELEPHONE : 01529 306 851

Information on qualified yoga teachers anywhere in the UK.

~~~

CANCER CARE SOCIETY,
21 ZETLAND ROAD,
REDLAND,
BRISTOL, BS6 7AH.

Offers trained counsellors and a national network of branches.

~~~

CANCER LINK,
17 BRITANNIA STREET,
LONDON, WC1X 9JN.
TELEPHONE : 0171 833 245

Information booklets and a directory of cancer support groups.

~~~

CANCER LINK,
9 CASTLE TERRACE,
EDINBURGH, EH1 2DP.
TELEPHONE : 0131 288 5557

CANCER RELIEF MACMILLAN FUND,
15 - 19 BRITTEN STREET,
LONDON, SW3 3TZ.
TELEPHONE : 0171 351 7811

Financial help in the form of grants to cancer patients and their families for hospital travel, heating bills and other special needs. They are also the source of the Macmillan specially trained home-care nurses.

~~~

COUNCIL FOR COMPLEMENTARY AND ALTERNATIVE MEDICINE,
SUITE 1, 19A CAVENDISH SQUARE,
LONDON, W1M 9AD.
TELEPHONE : 0171 724 9103

~~~

HOSPICE INFORMATION SERVICE,
51-59 LAWRIE PARK RD.,
SYDENHAM,
LONDON, SE26 6DZ.
TELEPHONE : 0181 778 9252

A directory of hospices plus information about home care and hospital support teams established throughout the UK and Eire.

~~~

IMPOTENCE INFORMATION CENTRE,
P O BOX 1130,
LONDON, W3 0BB.

~~~

ICSG,
INTERSTITIAL CYSTITIS SUPPORT GROUP,
13 HAZELWOOD ROAD,
NORTHAMPTON. NN1 1LG.

~~~

INTERNATIONAL STRESS MANAGEMENT ASSOCIATION,
THE PRIORY HOSPITAL,
PRIORY LANE,
LONDON, SW15 5JJ.
TELEPHONE : 0181 876 8261

~~~

IRISH CANCER SOCIETY,
5 NORTHUMBERLAND ROAD,
DUBLIN 4.
TELEPHONE : 01 681855

~~~

MARIE CURIE CANCER CARE,
28 BELGRAVE SQUARE,
LONDON, SW1X 8QG.
TELEPHONE : 0171 235 3325

Support and help to patients, with a range of residential nursing-homes and specialised home-nursing service.

~~~

NATURE'S BEST,
1 LAMBERTS ROAD,
TUNBRIDGE WELLS,
KENT, TN2 3EQ.
TELEPHONE : 01892 539595

This company operates a mail order service for over 150 nutritional supplements, one of them is Prostex a combination product, part of the ingredient is saw palmetto, used for the treatment of BPH. Prostex is not sold or recommended by Nature's Best in any way for the treatment of prostate cancer. The reason it is mentioned here is because it contains Beta-sitosterol.

~~~

PAIN ASSOCIATION SCOTLAND,
CRAMOND HOUSE,
CRAMOND GLEBE RD,
EDINBURGH, EH4 6NS.
TELEPHONE : 0131 312 7955

~~~

PAIN CONCERN (UK),
PO BOX 318,
CANTERBURY,
KENT, CT4 5DP.
TELEPHONE : 01227 26 677
(THE PHONE IS MANNED FROM 10am-4pm WEEKDAYS)

~~~

P.H.A.,
LANGWORTH,
LINCOLN, LN3 5DF.

The Prostate Help Association is a registered charity. It produces a quarterly Newsletter, not a glossy about fund raising events and how well the PHA workers are coping with the work load, but packed with relevant, some times controversial, comment on prostate operations and treatments ETC.. The PHA has no grants from government sources and depends almost entirely on subscriptions for its income. As well as informing men about the prostate condition it is also attempting to educate the great British public about the condition. (Send 2 x first class stamps for an initial information sheet and detail of the subscriptions and Support Network).

~~~

(SHIP). SELF HELP IN PAIN,
33 KINGSDOWN PARK,
TANKERTON,
KENT, CT5 2DT
TELEPHONE : 01227 264 677

~~~

SUE RYDER FOUNDATION,
CAVENDISH,
SUDBURY,
SUFFOLK, CO10 8AY.
TELEPHONE : 01787 280 252

They run care-homes for cancer patients.

~~~

TENOVUS,
COLLEGE BUILDINGS,
COURTENAY ROAD,
SPLOTTLANDS,
CARDIFF, CF2 2JP.
TELEPHONE : 01222 497700 ADMINISTRATION
0800 526 527   CANCER HELPLINE.

Support and information on any aspect of cancer. Prevention, screening, treatment, care, support services, personal & family problems, including welfare rights, benefits and legal issues, counselling, bereavement support. 9 am - 5 pm Monday to Friday.

~~~

ULSTER CANCER FOUNDATION,
40 - 42 EGLANTINE AVE
BELFAST, BT9 6DX
TELEPHONE 01232 663 439

For general interest.

The Edgar Cayce Centre,
13 Prospect Terrace,
New Kyo,
Stanley,
Co. Durham. DH9 7TR.
TELEPHONE : 01207 237696

USEFUL BOOKS TO READ.

There must be hundreds of books on cancer. So they will not all be listed here. Those that are will certainly lead you on to others if you want them. You will see as you progress that there are books to teach you to meditate, to massage, to visualize and books about vitamin and diet regimes. I would recommend the following to begin with :-.

The Bristol Experience　　　　　**ISBN 0 09 178980 X**

Mind Over Cancer　　　　　　　**ISBN 0 572 01451 1**

Cancer Help　　　　　　　　　　**ISBN 0 7459 2757 2**

Cancer - A Family Affair　　　　**ISBN 0 85969 706 1**

The Complete Book of Mens' Health ISBN 0 7225 3019 6

LETTERS FROM MEN AND THEIR WIVES.

Mr. J.....

I first consulted my GP in early summer 1993 about persistent pain in my ribs area, and thorough examinations and x-rays eliminated cracked ribs and serious chest/lung infections. However probably because I had a cough and had been down with pleurisy during the previous winter months, I was prescribed antibiotics - first Penicillin and two weeks later Ciprofloxacin, but my condition did not improve.

I began to feel rather anxious by mid-August as, prior to my becoming unwell, I was due for a trip to the USA for the whole of September and a decision was imminent as to whether or not I should cancel. However, I managed to convince myself there was some improvement, and, provided with a precautionary supply of antibiotics and painkillers by my GP, decided not to cancel.

The first two painful weeks in the US exhausted my supply of antibiotics, and I was obliged to seek the help and advice of a doctor in Canada. I explained my problems and pointed out that I was now experiencing pain throughout the whole of my upper skeletal frame; further examination and x-rays again confirmed no fractures, and it was concluded that 'pains were probably due to friction between rib bones and lungs' - again indicating the possibility of inflammation of the pleura. Back to square one ! Another course of Ciprofloxacin was prescribed, together with painkillers (which at a cost of about £65 seemed much less effective than those prescribed by my GP !) but which in the short term at least assisted in making me feel better for having 'done something'.

Sadly, however, there was no improvement in my condition and on my somewhat relieved return home two weeks later 4th October, my GP arranged to refer me to a consultant, meanwhile prescribing Naproxen tablets to counteract any joint inflammation. Two per day helped me feel a little better, but I would have been rather more reluctant to take them had I then known they also contained a pain killer. My Consultant arranged for me to undergo on 23rd Nov. what he described as a "special" x-ray examination which involved a radioactive isotope injection followed some hours later by a series of x-rays of my upper torso, and as a result of this, the Consultants assistant informed me on the 15th. December that the x-rays had shown up what he described as a serious bone abnormality, emanating from a malignant tumor 'somewhere' in my body, and in all probability despite the non-existence of the usual symptoms, that somewhere would prove to be my prostate gland. He went on to inform me that a blood test followed by a biopsy would be necessary to confirm the diagnosis, to which end I was referred to a consultant Urologist, who carried out these extra tests on a hospital day-visit on 29th Dec. The diagnosis was confirmed. And I was given two treatment options (1) testicular surgery or (2) hormonal type implants to be administered every 28 days. I opted for the implant treatment and received the first on the 20th January, together with 84 Cryproterone tablets taken over the first two weeks.

To date I have received two 3.6 mg implants of Zoladex at the hospital, I am an otherwise very fit 68 year old, and am pleased to say the treatment is already making life much easier for me, although the pains are not entirely eliminated. I find that with careful rest periods I can now manage without reverting to constant use of painkillers and my doctors prognosis is optimistic. I elected to discontinue taking Naproxen some time ago and am relieved I did so, as it appears that one side effect sometimes manifests itself in asthmatic-like symptoms... something of which I am aware, unfortunately at present........"

The letter is reproduced almost entirely because it shows that men have to be alert of changes in their bodies. It also allows us to glimpse a little of the trauma not of being diagnosed, but of **not** being diagnosed. One would like to think that if rectal and PSA screening had been available, Mr. J's condition would have been detected earlier.

Mrs B asks if the system is all that it should be !!

I am not at all happy with the investigations which were carried out prior to diagnosis. It is about 2 years since our GP picked up in a blood test a fault. My husband was told to return again 6 months later, for a further blood test. This was supposed to have been normal. However, a few months later my husband thought all was not well and returned to his GP to be given another test. This was once more not normal. Told to go back 3 months later for a further test, and still not normal, was referred to hospital. Waited for appointment with consultant another 2 months. Further tests lasting 3 months at least. By now having leg and joint pains in hips. After tests including bone scan was told he had bone cancer from the prostate gland.

His treatment was monthly injections in the stomach to shrink the gland, after 3 injections pains went. A further bone scan 6 months later and he was told his bones were just the same and his blood normal. Approx. 10 days later pains started and progressed for a further three months, still on injections and was finally sent for a one off radio-therapy course. This has helped the pain for the time being, but been given tablets which make him feel ill.

I am so annoyed at the fact it was found so soon and nothing was done for all that time. We did not know at first what was wrong with the blood. Had we known we would have pressed for further investigations much sooner, if it had been possible. The whole thing took too long.

Our hobby was walking, our whole lifestyle has been ruined. I am very bitter, my husband is 67, and only just retired.

~~~

Maybe Mrs B's letter will stimulate others out there to take a positive step, instead of hoping the medical profession will lead. Remember you are one person in a chattering crowd. You may have to shout to get heard. Shout louder !

Mrs F.

The prostate cancer my husband had suffered from since May 1994 spread rapidly during the spring and early summer into all his bones until he was unable to do anything for himself - not even move from his chair. Sadly he lost his fight against the disease and died early in July. I only wish we had known about PSA testing 2 years ago.

Mrs. D

My husband has recently been diagnosed as having prostate cancer and is undergoing hormone treatment with possibly radiotherapy at a later stage. Naturally this was a great shock to us as he had no symptoms and the cancer was discovered following a routine PSA test.

Mr. L.

In September 1988 I went to my GP with what I thought was lumbago plus cloudy urine. I was told it was a road accident I had had 17 years previously which at the time had meant a week off work, and had been the last time I had visited my GP.

The GP persisted with this diagnosis for some fifteen months, even at one time saying, "I cannot understand it". In December 1990 I changed GP's in the hope that it would bring about some action but the original policy was persisted with until 18 months later and after some aggressive behaviour on my part a TURP operation was undertaken on the 3rd. June 1991.

Four days after the operation the ward sister said the surgeon who had done the operation would like to speak to me regarding cancer. The shock on being told in the two minute interview, spoken in broken English, left me in a traumatic state.

Mr. C

I suffered prostate trouble for over a year with only tablets prescribed by my GP. He was very reluctant for me to have surgery, in the end I was so uncomfortable that I saw another doctor, who referred me to a consultant urologist. Within 10 days of seeing him he had performed a TURP, the pathology report showed that I had a small growth. I had 10 treatments of radiotherapy about three months ago. However I now find that returning to normal sex life is proving rather difficult.

Mr. F

After many months wait I had a TURP and was told all was well after a biopsy. Four years later I was back at square one with the same problems. The second TURP showed I had cancer and a scan confirmed it had spread to my bone. I was put on flutamide and told radiation was out of the question in my case but I could get no further information about the side effects of the tablets from the consultant. The tablets where changed to cyprostat because the side effects proved too severe to stand. These tablets have changed me completely so I had a word with my pharmacist. If I had know what they were doing to me I would never have agreed to such treatment as my doctor eventually agreed it was a chemical castration. I have never felt so ill. I think it is very sad that I have to write this letter at all. Why can't doctors be honest with their patients and save a lot of anxiety ?

Mr. B.

My cancer was found by accident. I was referred to a surgeon because I complained of an ache in my left groin. A hernia was suspected and confirmed after a two month wait for the appointment with the surgeon. I also mentioned my prostate problem and he gave me an internal examination and sent me for a scan and blood tests. This led to the cancer being discovered.

I take cyprostat, and after a few dizzy spells at first I feel fine but my lips have dried up, I am short of breath and get tired a lot easier.

Mr. T

After cancer was diagnosed I had an orchidectomy and cyprostat tablets. A scan had revealed a spread to the bone, my PSA level is still up at around 90 after a year of treatment. I find the medics are not forthcoming in advice on my future. But I have the feeling that my condition is incurable.

MRS. M.

In February 1995 my husband started getting bad indigestion, feeling sick, pain in groin on passing water and getting up 3 or 4 times a night. His prostate was never in question and he eventually went for a kidney xray in June. Two weeks later the urologist told us he had advanced prostate cancer possibly also in the bones. It was a total shock as my husband is only 58. He was put on a course of cyprostat tablets followed by monthly hormonal injections.

A bone scan in July revealed a 'hot spot' in his neck but no activity in his spinal area. The urologist said maybe no cancer in bones. Sent for neck xray. In August saw oncologist who really has nothing to say and hasn't even got the results of the July xray. She just read out what the urologist had said on our last visit. Ask our doctor to find out what was on the xrays..... he has no joy.

September find PSA now 4.5 and told it had been over 100.

November see oncologist who says keep on injections- when pressed she says cancer may become resistant to them - when pressed further finally produces results of xrays taken 4 months before - 'hot spot' in neck turns out to be wear and tear. So we have had 4 months worry for nothing.

My husband feels fine and has never had any pain. We really need to know what we are up against. Is there anybody out there who specialises in prostate cancer? After a urologist who is abrupt and with no bedside manner and an oncologist who does not want to give out any information, it would be nice to hear somebody talk sensibly.

~~~

It was letters like this which stimulated the writing of this book.

MR. Y.

After suffering with an enlarged prostate for over 10 years I had a TURP and six weeks after the operation visit my GP for a clearance to return to work. He advised me that the operation had shown a growth, I asked if this was cancer and he said yes ! His replies to my questions were brief and not encouraging. I can only think he did not know how to deal with the situation. I suffered severe shock and convinced myself that perhaps I had only six months to live. I left my job and started a course of radiotherapy, with thankfully no side effects. Eventually after many checkups I was told I was clear.

I have only one complaint to make. Following the radiotherapy treatment I was asked "Could I obtain an erection and did I still have intercourse ?" The answer was yes for about 2 months following the therapy and then quite suddenly I was impotent. I ask myself "why did they not advise me of the almost certain result of the treatment before I made the decision.?" It would not have made any difference to my decision to go ahead, but they should have explained.

Mr. E

I was very inadequately informed about my cancer prognosis, forms of treatment, side effects, symptoms etc.

My experience was that whilst the medics at all levels would readily respond to any specific question I posed, they themselves showed no desire to communicate with me on their own initiative. I had a distinct feeling they could not appreciate my deep need to be informed generally about my condition, to them I was merely 'the patient' , a job of work for them. Since I had an orchidectomy I have put on a stone in weight but having got all this trauma behind me, I have enjoyed excellent health, feel fine, have a good appetite and at 78 am active and cheerful, life is good.

The PHA receive hundreds of letters each month. I want to thank all those who write with their personal stories. Some are printed in the Newsletters. Perhaps the writers don't know just how much they help others who are following along in their footsteps.

If not, this is just to tell them that they do, a great deal.

(Philip Dunn)

—A—

acupuncture, 49
adrenal, 39
aneuploid, 23
Asian, 12, 55, 57, 59

—B—

Bacup, 29, 76
Beta-sitosterol, 54, 55
BIOPSY, 22
bladder instability, 36
BMJ, British Medical Journal, 18, 20, 21, 30
BPH, 8, 13, 17, 19, 34, 35, 36, 46, 52, 54, 55, 74

—C—

Cayce, 58
CHEMOTHERAPY, 43
Chinese, 12
Citizens Advice Bureau, 49
Corporal Jones, 19
CRYOTHERAPY, 35
CT, 23
cyproterone, 40, 47.
cystitis, 36
CYSTOSCOPY, 22

—D—

DHT, 13, 39, 51, 53, 55, 59
diarrhoea, 36
diet, 12
diploid, 23
DNA, 23, 57, 72
DRE, 8, 11, 14, 16, 17, 25

—E—

endorphins, 62
EPIC, 58

—F—

flare, 47
flare up, 40
FLOW RATE, 24,
flutamide, 40, 41, 71
free floating PSA, 20

—G—

Gerson, 60
Gleason, 27

—H—

HIFU, 35
hormonal, 67
hormone, 26, 39, 40, 56, 68, 69
hypnotherapy, 49

—I—

impotence, 17, 34, 67
impotent, 33, 41
incontinence, 17, 33, 34, 67
infertility, 17, 34, 67

—L—

Lancet, 20, 54, 57, 58
LAPAROSCOPIC LYMPH NODE DISSECTION, 32
lymph, 23, 25, 71
lymph nodes, 9
lymphatic, 45
lymphatic system, 8

—M—

MAB, 27, 37, 41, 42, 71
macrobiotic, 61
MARIMASTAT, 42, 43
metastases, 26
metastatic, 42, 45
Metastron, 47
MICROWAVE, 35
morphine, 46
MR (I), 23

—N—

nausea, 36, 45, 46

—O—

oestrogens, 55
oncologist, 46
orchidectomy, 26, 39, 40

—P—

PAP, 21
PHA, 8, 11, 20, 76
PIN, 18, 51, 52, 68
pituitary, 40
POSITIVE THINKING, 61
Proscar, 13, 19, 51, 52
Prostabrit, 54, 73
Prostap, 40
Prostex, 54
PSA, 11, 14, 15, 16, 18, 19, 20, 71

—R—

RACIAL, 12
RAD Magazine, 19, 23, 37
radiation, 37, 47, 67
radical prostatectomy, 26, 32, 33, 37
Radiotherapy, 26, 27, 33, 36, 39, 42, 46, 62, 68
Reflexology, 49
retrograde ejaculation, 7

—S—

Sabel serrulata, 54
saw palmetto, 54, 73
secondaries, 45
sexual activity, 11
sphincter, 26
sphincter muscles, 7
stiboestrol, 39, 40
Suprefact, 40
Suramin, 43
Swedes, 12

—T—

Tenovus, 29, 76
testicles, 13
testosterone, 13, 39, 40, 41, 42, 52, 73

TRUS, 11, 21
TURAPY, 34, 35
TURP, 7, 33, 37

—U—

URINE ANALYSIS, 17

—V—

venereal disease, 11
visualization, 62, 64
vitamin D, 58
vitamins, 61

—W—

watchful waiting', 14, 15, 23, 32, 67
WDDTY, 28, 58, 60

—Y—

yoga, 65

—Z—

Zoladex, 40, 41, 71

Decode

Cut out and use as a book mark

BPH (Non cancerous prostate enlargement)

CT (A body scan)

DHT (Testosterone after it has been converted)

DRE (Digital Rectal Examination).

HIFU (High-Intensity Focused Ultrasound)

IMPOTENCE (Inability to achieve an erection)

MAB (Maximum Androgen Blockade)

MRI (A body scan)

PAP (A blood test which checks for cancer)

PHA (Prostate Help Association)

PIN (A pre cancer state of prostate tissue)

PSA (A blood test which checks for cancer)

TRUS (Trans-Rectal Ultrasound)

TURAPY (An out-patient treatment to remove obstructive prostate tissue)

TURP...(An operation to remove obstructive prostate tissue).